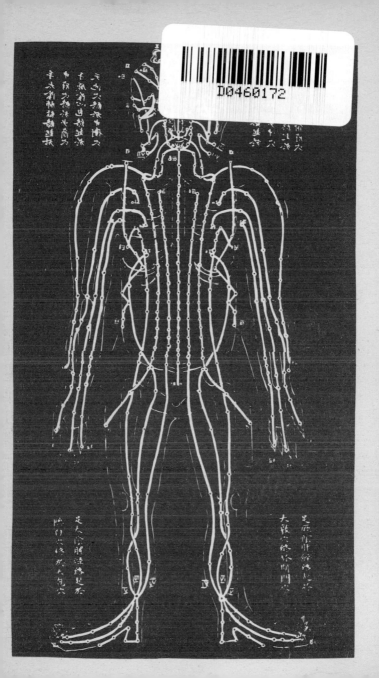

MENTOR Titles of Related Interest

Chinese Folk Medicine

by Heinrich Wallnöfer
and Anna von Rottauscher

Translated by Marion Palmedo

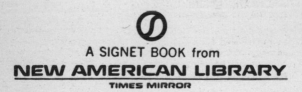

A SIGNET BOOK from
NEW AMERICAN LIBRARY
TIMES MIRROR

SIGNET TRADEMARK REG. U.S. PAT. OFF. AND FOREIGN COUNTRIES
REGISTERED TRADEMARK—MARCA REGISTRADA
HECHO EN CHICAGO, U.S.A.

SIGNET, SIGNET CLASSICS, SIGNETTE, MENTOR AND PLUME BOOKS
are published by The New American Library, Inc.,
1301 Avenue of the Americas, New York, New York 10019

FIRST PRINTING, January, 1972

PRINTED IN THE UNITED STATES OF AMERICA

PUBLISHER'S NOTE

CHINESE FOLK MEDICINE contains many treatments and alleged cures that have been used in China for centuries. In this volume the ingredients, recipes, and remedies are printed just as they have been handed down from one generation to another in China. No attempt has been made to check these medically; no reader should assume that any cure in this book has been approved and may be used without further investigation.

CONTENTS

FOREWORD

A new world is opening up before us, a world abounding in symbolism and mystic images, but rich also in genuine knowledge of man's living and dying.

Anyone who is not familiar to some extent with the Chinese concept of the universe is likely to insist on seeing merely superstition and witchcraft in the medical practices of the Chinese and in their theories about the structure and function of the human body. That, however, does an injustice to the ancient culture of the East and its achievements. It means showing as much prejudice as did the "conquerors" of only a few generations ago, when they tried to force upon the Chinese the often rather doubtful blessings of Western civilization. Books written as recently as the turn of the century still speak condescendingly of the "foolish, unfounded superstition" to be encountered in the East. In the meantime, some of that superstition has been proven to be of substantial value; much of it is still waiting to be elucidated. But we are by no means justified in discarding the wisdom of the East as nonsense merely because microscope and atom bomb were invented by the "white race."

In the West today, the autonomous nervous system with its two opposing-balancing forces is generally known and recognized, and it serves excellently to demonstrate the relationship between the concepts of East and West. It is for this reason that we introduce the theory of *Yin* and *Yang*—which might be considered the Eastern counterpart to the nervous system—at the beginning of our book. Our work does not profess to be either a textbook or a comprehensive collection of Chinese medical practices; its intention is to arouse a desire among laymen, as well as the professional world, to become better acquainted with a complex system of ideas that is new and foreign to us. To this day, millions of people in China and Japan are being treated by native Chinese medical methods—methods that are often less successful, but at the right times probably more successful, than ours. And if for no other reason than that, the study of Chinese medicine deserves our attention. Perhaps our book will also help to put the concepts of both worlds into their proper place of value and importance.

Today's over-specialization, for instance, which is commented on profusely by many modern physicians, is not such a recent phenomenon as they would have us believe. If, as claimed, the twentieth-century doctor has lost the personal touch with his patient, then perhaps we should find consolation in the fact that about 450 years before our era, the Greek historian Herodotus deplored the dilemma of medical specialization in Egypt. And undoubtedly it was over-specialization that also froze the acupuncture and pulse theories of the Chinese into the rigid molds in which they are found today and which make them appear so alien to us.

There is much well-observed truth in the ancient Chinese medical writings. But it is as well to remember that the Chinese always did—and still do—consider meditation far more valuable than experiment, the image more significant than the object. Assuming that the saying "Experiment is the mother of science" represents the thesis of the West, we might say that the East holds to its antithesis: Meditation is the father of science.

We, too, recognize symbolism. But we are far less entangled with it than the peoples of the Far East in whose theaters, for example, each finger movement bears a symbolic significance. The symbols of the Chinese, the correspondences between all parts of the cosmos, are a most essential part of Chinese philosophy and medicine. We therefore open our book with an explanation of these correspondences.

For the student of the Chinese language, we should like to add that internationally accepted terminology has been used throughout. Anyone who is at all aware of the complexities of Chinese writing will realize how difficult it can be to interpret an expression correctly. Indeed, in many instances, a "correct" interpretation does not exist. The translator either has to depend on oral traditions, or resort to his own intuition.

I

THE FUNDAMENTALS

OF CHINESE MEDICINE

Any attempt at probing into the nature of Chinese medicine must begin with a search into the age-old philosophy from which it sprang—from which, indeed, all Eastern concepts and knowledge of illness, of cure, and of death evolved. For the complex of Eastern thinking is so far removed from the modern Western mind that we often lack the very words in which to express certain Eastern concepts. True, we are confronted here with a distant oriental culture, but that alone does not explain the gap. The crucial difference lies in the overall mental attitude toward nature and life—an attitude more akin to the beliefs and concepts of Europe of the Middle Ages.

The "Tao"

The first step, then, is to search for the *tao* (in the monosyllabic Old Chinese, pronounced somewhat like "dow"). The accurate translation of *tao* has troubled Western scholars throughout history, for no other language possesses a word that can render fully all the connotations and subtle overtones of this *tao*. In daily usage, *tao means* "way," "path," also "discourse." But on a more spiritual level it symbolizes the absolute Way of nature, the primeval law that regulates all heavenly and earthly matters. Chinese scholars found this expression for it:

The way that can be mapped is not the eternal Way.
The name that can be named is not the eternal Name.

These are the opening words of the *Tao Tê Ching,* the great classic of the Chinese mystics. In its twenty-fifth

11

chapter, Lao-tzu, to whose authorship the book is attributed, sings of the *tao* thus:

> Something there is, whose veiled creation was
> Before the earth or sky began to be;
> So silent, so aloof and so alone,
> It changes not, nor fails, but touches all:
> Conceive it as the mother of the world.
> I do not know its name;
> A name for it is "Way";
> Pressed for designation,
> I call it Great.
> Great means outgoing,
> Outgoing, far-reaching,
> Far-reaching, return.*

"You may rest within the *tao,* but you cannot define it," said the philosopher Chuang-tzu.

To live according to the *tao* means to adapt oneself to the order of nature and to pursue a mode of life in concord with the Ultimate Principle. Chinese medical works speak with reverence of the sages of ancient times who knew of the Way and "led their lives in *tao.*"

The Correspondences

In Chinese cosmology, the universe is conceived of as a vast indivisible entity. Within it, each single being has its definite function. No one thing can exist without the others, and to each thing, in turn, is linked a chain of concepts which correspond to each other in harmonious balance. To violate this harmony is to hurl chaos, wars and catastrophes upon all mankind, and sickness upon the individual. Man must therefore strive to adjust himself wholly within the world of those "correspondences," in which the five elements—wood, fire, earth, metal, and water—constitute the guiding principles. These are said to create one another, but also destroy one another, depending on the sequence of enumeration.

> Wood creates fire.
> Fire creates earth.

* From *The Way of Life* by Lao Tzu, translated by R. B. Blakney, © 1955 by Raymond B. Blakney, New American Library, Inc., New York City.

Earth creates metal.
Metal creates water.
Water creates wood.

Wood destroys earth.
Earth destroys water.
Water destroys fire.
Fire destroys metal.
Metal destroys wood.

Since these basic tenets also define the structure of Chinese medicine, it is essential that we become familiar with at least some of the interpretations of these producing-vanquishing processes.

Creation:

Wood creates fire:	Two pieces of wood rubbed together produce sparks.
Fire creates earth:	Fire transforms burning matter into ashes.
Earth creates metal:	Within the earth, ore is "born."
Metal creates water:	Melting metal becomes liquid.
Water creates wood:	Through being watered the tree grows.

Destruction:

Wood destroys earth:	The tree sucks strength from the earth.
Earth destroys water:	Earth can halt the flow of water (also: earth soaks up water).
Water destroys fire:	Water extinguishes the flame.
Fire destroys metal:	Fire causes metal to melt.
Metal destroys wood:	The ax fells the tree.

Closely associated with these elements are the five planets Jupiter, Mars, Saturn, Venus and Mercury. Chinese belief endows these planets with qualities that in some respects differ significantly from those of Western astrology.

Jupiter:	Planet of magnanimity and gentleness.
Mars:	Pioneer and instigator.
Saturn:	Planet of natural dignity and authority.
Venus:	Planet of sensuous enjoyment, but also of wars and of jurisdiction.
Mercury:	Planet of intelligence, of dangers, but also of retreat.

The following table serves to demonstrate how these elements and planets are correlated to still other images and concepts. Here compiled are those correspondences that are most pertinent to the Chinese theory of the cosmos.

THE CORRESPONDENCES

EMOTION	Anger	Joy	Sorrow	Fear	Compassion
FLUID	Tears	Perspiration	Mucus	Saliva	—
TISSUES	Ligaments	Arteries	Skin & Hair	Bones	Muscles
ORIFICES	Eyes	Ears	Mouth	Genitals	Nose
VISCERA	Liver	Heart	Lungs	Kidneys	Spleen
FLAVOR	Sour	Bitter	Tart	Salty	Sweet
CLIMATE	Wind	Heat	Dryness	Cold	Humidity
COLOR	Green	Red	White	Black	Yellow
GUIDING RULES OF BEHAVIOR FOR HIGH OFFICIALS	Exercise Mildness	Instigate	Sit in Judgment	Retreat	Contemplate
PLANETS	Jupiter	Mars	Venus	Mercury	Saturn
ELEMENTS	Wood	Fire	Metal	Water	Earth
TIME OF DAY	Morning	Noon	Evening	Night	—
CHARACTER OF SEASON	Blossoming	Ripening	Harvesting	Storing	Preserving
SEASON	Spring	Summer	Autumn	Winter	Late Summer— Early Autumn
RULERS OVER THE DIRECTIONS	Green Dragon	Red Bird	White Tiger	Turtle. Black Warrior	—
WORLD DIRECTION	East	South	West	North	Center

If man wishes to remain healthy, he must attune himself and his actions to conform with this ever moving cycle. To achieve this, precise instructions were given in such historical works as the *Lü Chih Ch'un Ch'iu* (the *Spring and Autumn Annals* by Lü Pu Wei, who died around 230 B.C.), from which the following directives for the emperor and his highest officials are taken. A comparison with the table of Correspondences will illustrate how rigidly the basic laws were pursued.

"During the three spring months, the emperor remains in the eastern wing of the Hall of Light [the principal building for cult rituals]. He rides in a carriage drawn by green-shimmering dragon-horses. All the banners are green. His officials and entourage are dressed in green gowns and wear green jade jewelry. The emperor conducts the sacrificial rites on the palace's east lawn. He orders his ministers to be magnanimous and to exercise gentleness, and to prevent the felling of trees and the taking up of arms [wood is destroyed by metal!].

"During the three summer months, the emperor confines himself to the southern wing of the Hall of Light. His carriage is scarlet and is drawn by fox-red horses. The banners are red. The emperor's staff are clad in red robes and wear red jade. Sacrificial rites are conducted on the south lawn. The emperor orders his ministers to nominate worthy persons for awards and medals and to urge the populace to apply themselves to their tasks with vigor.

"During the last days of the summer season, the emperor remains in the central chambers of the Hall of Light. He rides a carriage drawn by dun-colored horses. The banners are yellow. His entourage is dressed in yellow and wears yellow jade jewelry. The emperor observes the sacrificial rites in the central temple.

"During the three autumn months, the emperor stays in the western wing of the Hall of Light. His war-carriage is drawn by white horses. The banners are white. His officials wear white gowns and white jade jewels. He conducts sacrificial rites on the palace's west lawn. The emperor orders his ministers to revise the laws and to conduct the court trials. Dressed in his war habit, the emperor personally takes part in the hunting expeditions.

"During the three winter months, the emperor confines himself to the north wing of the Hall of Light. He rides a black carriage drawn by black horses. The banners are black. His staff wear black robes and black jade. Sacrificial rites are observed on the north lawn. The emperor orders his ministers to replenish the storage vaults and to have all necessary repairs done on doors and locks. On the eve of the New Year, the exorcisers are called for to expel the spirits of pestilence."

"Yin" and "Yang"

In the shadow of his small, broad-gabled house sat Ling Ch'i, the physician. His eyes wandered eagerly over the complicated, often indistinct brush strokes in the ancient book, *Huang-ti nei ching*. Even at his time—Ling Ch'i lived around 1000 B.C.—this work was already a venerable old book of wisdom from the long past days of the Chou Dynasty.

More and more fascinating grew the reading. The book told of things wondrous and unbelievable. A stream, it said, flows through the human body, an eternally pulsing red sap; and indeed, Ling Ch'i himself had often seen this red fluid when a careless person had injured himself. But the book went on to say that there were two kinds of blood. In one kind, *Yin* was prevailing, the principle of day; in the other, *Yang*, the principle of night. In spite of his admiration for the ancient teacher, Ling Ch'i could not help smiling when he laid the book aside. All due respect to the eminent master's wise opinions—he evidently knew well what he meant by these written characters—but he, Ling Ch'i, was too insignificant to aspire to such a lofty flight of thought. Why should he let the teachings of *Huang-ti nei ching* confuse his life?

If Ling Ch'i had been forced to hang a lantern in front of his door for every patient who died in his practice—as his colleagues were forced to do hundreds of years later—the number of his dead would have been no smaller and no larger than theirs.

Huang-ti nei ching (*The Yellow Emperor's Book of Internal Medicine*) is the first work known to contain any suggestion of knowledge of the circulation of the blood, which was to be next recognized almost 4,000 years later. Like Ling Ch'i, all Chinese physicians have read the teachings of the great master who conceived of a circulatory system thousands of years ago, who could already distinguish the oxygen-starved blood of the veins from the life-giving blood of the arteries, and who divined their correlation to the two basic world principles, *Yin* and *Yang*.

In the Western world, it is quite conceivable to practice medicine without an underlying philosophy and religion. Even a confirmed unbeliever or an adversary to any philosophical thinking can be an accomplished surgeon. This, of course, was not always true in the West; but in the medical world of the East it is utterly inconceivable. Heaven and earth, gods and demons are so tightly interwoven with the human being that medical treatment without proper knowledge of cosmic relationships becomes impossible. This accounts for the very early appearance in history of the intense study and evaluation of the weather, the seasons, the stars and the course of the moon. Also, the fact that long before our era Chinese physicians were essentially aware of the function and significance of the nerves can be traced back to their doctrine of man as an integral part of the universe. And on the ensuing concept of an eternal duality, of positive and negative, stimulator and preserver, light and shadow, day and night, and on the recognition that they are of equal value and that one cannot exist without the other—on these were erected the very pillars of Chinese philosophy.

Yin and *Yang* are the primordial twin potencies that regulate the universe, and they have bestowed power onto all the "ten thousand things" within that universe. *Yang* represents the male, positive energy, producing light, warmth, and fullness. *Yin* is female, "negative," the force of darkness, of the cold, and of emptiness. As *Yin* and *Yang* manipulate heaven and earth in the waxing and waning of seasons and days, so they exert their power over the human being.

When the complex network of the autonomic nervous system was first discovered by medical science, it was assumed that it consisted of two strictly separated systems, functioning independently of each other. More recent research, however, has revealed that the nerve fibers of the sympathetic system—the "stimulator" among the nerves—are always accompanied by nerve ends of the parasympathetic system—the chief "preserver." This modern discovery must come to mind when we learn that *Yin* cannot be without *Yang*, nor *Yang* without *Yin*. "Within each *Yang* there exists *Yin*; within each *Yin* must be *Yang*," as the medical writings of Old China state.

Two Viennese physicians attained notable positions in the world of medicine when they set out to ascertain the crucial role that the autonomic nervous system plays in bringing about diseases. Yet, the *Nei Ching,* the oldest Chinese medical textbook, already teaches us that diseases occur when the

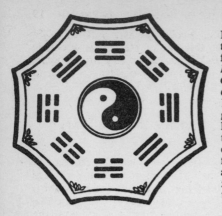

Fig. 1. The figure shows the eight Kua, trigrams from the ancient classic *I Ching* (*Book of Changes*), surrounding the elemental forces *Yin* and *Yang*. All of them together represent the evolution and eternal permutations of nature. In the center, *Yin* is perceived flowing into *Yang,* even as *Yang* approaches its zenith; while *Yang* begins to flow in, even as *Yin* is approaching its zenith.

balance between *Yin* and *Yang* is disturbed! And the book is even more explicit: "If *Yang* is predominant, then the body will grow hot; the pores close and the patient begins to breathe heavily and gasp for breath. Fever will arise; the palate will become dry; the person becomes tense and irritable." What is the modern diagnosis? The ever nervous busybody, the high-strung fellow who easily falls into quarrels, whose body temperature is constantly raised because of the faster burning-processes in his organism—he suffers from over-functioning of the thyroid gland. We also know that the sympathetic nerves play a significant part in this disease; and, indeed, many researchers hold that an over-functioning of the sympathetic "stimulator" is the cause of the over-functioning of the thyroid gland.

"If *Yin* and *Yang* are not in harmony, it is as though there were no autumn opposite the spring, no winter opposite the summer. When *Yin* and *Yang* part from each other, the strength of life wilts and the breath of life is extinguished. If such a body is exposed to the dew and the wind, then colds and fever will set in." Today we speak of the "predisposition" that makes it possible for germs to settle in the organism.

Of course, not every passage in Chinese medical works affords such obvious comparison; still, there is no lack of interesting connections. And so the *Nei Ching* continues: "There is also *Yin* within *Yin,* and *Yang* within *Yang.* Thus from early morn to the middle of day the *Yang* of Heaven is effective; this is the '*Yang* within *Yang.*' From midday until dusk, the *Yang* of Heaven is again effective, but now it is the 'Yin within Yang.' From the first dark of night until the cock's first crow, the Yin of Heaven is effective; this is the 'Yin within Yin.' From the cock's first crowing until the early morning hours, the Yin of Heaven is again effective, but now it is the 'Yang within Yin.' "

"Yin" and "Yang" and the Human Body*

The various parts of the human body likewise correspond to the dual principle of Yin and Yang. The body's surface is Yang, the inside is Yin. Yang is within the back part, Yin within the front part of the body. Yin is also the five Ts'ang-viscera—liver, heart, spleen, lungs and kidneys; the six Fu-bowels—gall bladder, stomach, large intestine, small intestine, bladder and "warmer"—are Yang. The diseases of winter and spring are in Yin, the diseases of summer and autumn in Yang.

> The heart is the Yang within Yang.
> The lungs are the Yin within Yang
> The liver is the Yang within Yin.
> The spleen is the Yin within Yin.

Also, the pulse is controlled by Yin and Yang. If one knows the Yang, one recognizes the Yin in the pulse accordingly; if one knows the Yin, one recognizes Yang.

Yin wants to turn inside; Yang seeks to thrust through to the outside and appears there as perspiration. The aura of Yang nourishes the mind and simultaneously influences the muscles. If it does not succeed in opening and closing the pores properly, the aura of coldness will set in; swellings will occur and later ulcers that will penetrate into the flesh. The aura in the blood vessels is weakened, and the patient seems inclined toward anxiety and fears. If the aura in the blood vessels is not in harmony with the condition of the flesh, ulcers and tumors will result; perspiration cannot be dispersed, the body wastes, the aura will melt away, and the "hollow points" (corresponding points, a term in acupuncture) will close up. If in addition Yang prevails, the patient will die of this over-accumulation. When the Yang aura is hemmed in, the compression has to be relieved immediately.

* For a full description of Chinese anatomy and physiology, see Chapter IV.

If this is not done to a sufficient degree, the *Yang* aura is destroyed. It is therefore essential that the *Yang* aura be shielded from damages, so that muscles and bones may not be endangered. He who exposes himself to dew or fog and pays no heed to the hours of the day will enervate his body. If *Yin* is too strong, the body will grow chilly and the patient will perspire incessantly. People of this type are nervous and apprehensive and catch colds easily. In time they will become rebellious and will eventually die of an overloading of the stomach. They may survive a summer, but not the winter. Such people should seek to avoid the "seven harms" and to exploit the "eight favors," and through them should try to establish a balance between *Yin* and *Yang*. If they do not accomplish this, their lives will be of short duration. Half of the *Yin* force has been used up at the age of forty. At fifty, the human body becomes sluggish; eyes no longer see; ears no longer hear. At sixty, the *Yin* force is exhausted, and deterioration sets in. The "nine orifices" are of little use any more: the lower ones are dry and empty; the upper ones are brim-full. Soon exhaustion is so complete that even tears can no longer flow.

But those who have striven for the ultimate wisdom in their lives retain unimpaired vision and hearing, and their bodies remain vigorous and lithe despite old age. He who does not strive for such wisdom ages very rapidly.

Yin is thought to store the vital strength of life (today's theory: the parasympathetic nervous system serves to build up the body; it controls the digestive processes and stores bodily reserves). *Yang* is said to protect the body from outside infiltrations and therefore must be maintained in stalwart condition. If *Yin* cannot match *Yang*, the pulse will faint away and the patient will become insane. If, on the other hand, *Yang* cannot match *Yin*, the auras of the five *Ts'ang*-viscera will be thrown into disorder, and circulation in the nine orifices will cease. The ancient sages, it is said, guarded the perfect balance of *Yin* and *Yang* jealously; thus their bones and marrow were strong and firm. They also adapted the breath and blood to the principles of the dual power, and their inner and outer organs performed in like harmony. Hence *Yin* and *Yang* could not be injured by evil influences.

If a *Yang* aura is not preserved sufficiently strong, the *Yin* aura will perish. But if *Yin* aura and *Yang* aura are sound and sane and living in peaceful interaction, then man's mind and body will be in proper order.

"Yin" and "Yang" and the Directions of the World

Heaven could not subsist on North and West alone, for North and West are *Yin*. And man, accordingly, sees and hears less well with his right eye and right ear than with his left eye and ear. The earth could not subsist on East and South alone, for East and South are *Yang*. Hence, man's left hand and left foot are less strong than his right ones.

The reason: East is the region where *Yang* dwells. The essences of *Yang* rise up to Heaven. Heaven is filled with light; on earth darkness reigns, and emptiness. This makes man's eye and ear keen, but hand and foot inadequate. West is the region of *Yin*. The essences of *Yin* sink down onto earth. Thus abundance rules below now, and emptiness above. This makes eye and ear inadequate, and hand and foot capable of functioning.

The Significance of Fever in Chinese Medicine

"His Excellency, Master Hsin, Chief Supervisor of the Imperial Storage Vaults, would be much obliged if you would have the kindness to pay him a visit." This request was brought one day before Tsang Kung the doctor. "For days now, His Excellency has struggled with a high fever, and none of the doctors who were sent for have been able to free him of it." Tsang Kung went to see the sick man. Standing at his bedside, he studied the patient's complexion for a while, then took his limp hand and began to examine his pulse.

"No reason for worry," he declared briefly, "the disease is not fatal. I believe Your Excellency has caught this heavy catarrh through contact with running cold water. The eruption of the fever can be due only to such a cause."

"It is exactly as you say," agreed the Chief Supervisor excitedly. "A very short while ago, I was sent to Ch'u by the Imperial Court. When I had reached Lu Hsien and was about to cross the bridge, my horse suddenly shied and I was thrown into the river. Naturally, I was pulled out of the water immediately, but my robes were soaked through.

When I finally arrived at Ch'u, my body was burning hot. Since then I have not been able to conquer this fever."

Dr. Tsang Kung prescribed a sudorific, a medicine to induce perspiration. The patient took it several times, whereupon the fever declined, and soon His Excellency was fully recovered.

THE SIX REGIONS AND FEVER

For the clinician of today—with the exception perhaps of a few sages of internal medicine—laboratory reports and chemical examinations are of paramount value. Not so for the Old Chinese physicians; but then, they were undisputed masters in the art of observing the patient. To be sure, the conclusions they drew from their observations seem rather adventurous to modern minds. Moreover, they were probably larded with obscure allusions and instructions in order to mystify the "competition." But if we push through to their very core, some of these old writings will appear like Western textbooks of the nineteenth century, the golden age of objective patient-observation.

In the *Nei Ching,* for instance, we may find the following pronouncement: "Fever can generally be cured within ten days. If, however, the disease is of a severe nature, all the arts of medicine will be useless; death will occur after six or seven days."

The doctor of today will be reminded of his own experience when he reads further that higher fever does not necessarily indicate greater danger. How often has he not calmed down a mother who was terrified over her baby's hot little body. "Only when the five *Ts'ang*-viscera (liver, heart, spleen, lungs, kidneys) and the six *Fu*-bowels (gall bladder, stomach, large and small intestines, bladder and 'warmer') have been injured by the 'chill'—only then is death inevitable."

The fever's course through the three *Yin* and the three *Yang* regions is described in equal detail. On the first day, skin and body-hair (the region of *T'ai Yang*) are beset by the chill, headache will follow, and "the spine will grow stiff." Today's textbooks also cite shivers, gooseflesh, and aches in the joints as fever symptoms.

The second day brings pains in the eyes, the nose dries up, the patient becomes restless, and his body is glowing hot. "Small wonder," Chinese doctors would comment, "because on the second day the disease proceeds to the region of *Yang Ming*, the ruler of the flesh who is intricately connected with the nasal passages and the eyes."

On the third day, the disease advances into the region of *Shao Yang*, which presides over the gall bladder. The *Shao Yang* pulse leads into the ribs and up into the ear. Pains will therefore appear in chest and ribs (presumably the patient has pleurisy), and impaired hearing will result. The three *Yang* regions with their veins and arteries have thus absorbed the sickness, but it has not yet penetrated into the intestines. Heavy perspiration may still expel it.

And so through the following days of the fever. True to the principle of correspondences, the individual organs are now being attacked in successive order. The *T'ai Yin* region is attacked on the fourth day—*T'ai Yin* extends to the inside of the stomach and is closely connected with the larynx, which dries up; on the fifth day the *Shao Yin* region —its pulse reaches to the kidneys and is connected with the lungs and the root of the tongue, and so the patient is parched with thirst; and on the sixth day the *Chüeh Yin* region. *Chüeh Yin* stretches to the sexual organs and is connected with the liver; a distended stomach and lack of appetite are the result, as well as a distinct atrophy of the scrotum—today still recognized as a symptom of physical exhaustion. This sixth day bears the greatest danger, since all three *Yang* and all three *Yin* regions have now been seized by the raging fever. Circulation is slackening and will finally cease altogether; the patient expires.

If he was fortunate, however, and the five *Ts'ang*-viscera and the six *Fu* bowels were left unharmed, the disease may turn. Improvement will begin in the *T'ai Yang* region during the seventh day and the headache will subside (before the introduction of penicillin, that day marked the crisis in the course of pneumonia). The eighth day will find *Yang Ming* restored and the fever abated. On the ninth day the patient will begin to hear better, since *Shao Yang*, too, is recovering (in children, an inflammation of the middle ear frequently accompanies pneumonia). On the tenth day the bloated feeling in the stomach decreases and the appetite returns, for *T'ai Yin* is being revived. During the eleventh day the sensation of thirst disappears; the tongue loses its dryness; the patient has sneezing fits. *Shao Yin* is mending. On the twelfth day, finally, *Chüeh Yin* heals; the scrotum regains normal size, the breath loses its bad odor, and one day later the patient is restored to health.

What do the ancient teachers prescribe as treatment? Fasting, perspiring, strengthening of the circulation—"proper balance must be re-established among the inner organs." Should the fever persist for more than three days, their instructions are to ensure regular evacuation of the bowels.

What do modern doctors prescribe, aside from antibiotics? Fasting, laxatives, and sweat-inducing medicines, either natural ones (herbal teas) or chemical ones (aspirin).

Especially emphasized by Chinese doctors is fasting. Chronic defects, they say, may be attributed to rich food during the high-fever days. Although the disease itself has been dispelled, heat still lingers within the body. The breath mingles with the foodstuff until the heats of both are interlocked. Again, we are only left to wonder: Was it known to those ancient practitioners that we obtain our body warmth from the absorption of food?

A blunder over diet is not irretrievable. If the doctor recognizes deficiency and abundance in the body and appraises them judiciously, and if he then succeeds in reinstating the body's harmony, the patient may still recover. However, should he consume meat too soon, a relapse must be expected. And if, in fact, the meal was too plentiful, permanent damage may have been done.

One passage of the *Nei Ching* even anticipates a possible objection. One might protest, "When the chill (the fever) has already seized all of the inner organs, the circulation has stopped, and blood and life-forces are powerless, how can it be that the patient can live for three more days, and death strikes only then?" *Yang Ming* also governs the twelve main blood vessels and still possesses sufficient strength to prevent life's final escape, even though the sick person no longer recognizes anybody. But when three days have passed, even this strength is exhausted, and the patient "wanders beyond the four directions of the world."

II

THE EVOLUTION

OF CHINESE MEDICINE

The Emperor had left the audience hall and was returning to his chambers, on his face a bright smile of satisfaction. The ministers of agriculture had lavished their praises on the new farm implement. And the peasants, so they reported, had adopted the new tilling method with enthusiasm. The tool was his, the Emperor's, own invention: a wing-shaped iron structure with which the ground could be loosened and shoveled over very easily. Indeed, he had tried it with his own hands only a short while ago, and it had worked splendidly. But now his plough had passed its real test. And the Emperor's smile broadened.

At last, he could devote himself completely to his true passion—the study of the inner organs of the human body. For Heaven had endowed him with an extraordinary gift: a peephole into his stomach. The walls of his stomach and the skin over it were so thin and transparent that he could observe everything that took place inside it. What a fascinating pastime! All his life he had been captivated by the mysteries of medicine and had made the study of herb-remedies his special concern. In the end—what could be more natural?—he had begun to try out these herbs on his own body.

Thus, for one whole year now, he had swallowed a different plant each day and had studied its effect on his stomach. His reward had been the discovery of poisonous herbs, which he examined and finally rendered harmless by using certain antitoxins. Alas, the Emperor was not permitted to continue his research much longer; when he had concluded over seventy such experiments, death finally caught up with him. He died in the year 2697 B.C., at the age of 123 years. In appreciation of his merits, he was subsequently promoted into the realm of deities and was

25

awarded the title and epithet Emperor Shen Nung, Patron
God of Agriculture.

A more recent example of this medical oddity was the
Canadian Alexis H. Martin, who was afflicted with an "open
stomach" caused by a bullet wound. Nobody was willing to
employ this man until his physician, Dr. William Beaumont,
took him on as a servant. Henceforth, Mr. Martin served
his employer as an excellent guinea pig, while the doctor, in
turn, secured him a name in the annals and textbooks of
medicine. In 1833, Dr. Beaumont published the results of
his numerous thorough experiments in the treatise *Experiments and Observations on the Gastric Juice and the Physiology of Digestion.*

Huang-ti, The Yellow Emperor

Fire had been Shen Nung's patron element, for which he
was also called The Red Emperor. His successor, who is
said to have reigned from about 2697 to 2595 B.C., called
the earth his patron element. Thus, in deference to the
earth's color, he was named Huang-ti, The Yellow Emperor.
In wisdom and in thirst for knowledge he was in no way second to his predecessor. One day, inspired by the design of
the Great Dipper in the sky, he constructed a cart in its
image and mounted it on wheels. This attempt proved so
astoundingly successful that in the course of time he established a whole car park. Everyone stood in awe and admiration before this modern means of transportation. Soon after,
the Emperor erected a planetarium, in order that the course
of the planets might be observed more accurately. Not satisfied with these accomplishments, he began to work out a
system of musical tones and chords and then designed the
instruments on which to play them. And yet, the bulk of his
life's endeavor—aside from the introduction of a monetary
system—was directed toward the exploration of all aspects
of medicine. With his minister Ch'i Po he would enter into
heated debates revolving around the art of acupuncture, or
the influences of wind, heat, cold, and humidity on the human body. The celebrated *Nei Ching* is often ascribed to
him. However, many scholars now maintain that it was
probably not recorded on paper until the end of the Chou
Dynasty, which lasted from about 1100 to 250 B.C. Since
this book contains many translations from the *Nei Ching*, a
description of that ancient work is appropriate here.

The "Nei Ching"

The *Nei Ching* is composed of two main parts, the *Su wen* and the *Ling shu*. The first part, *Su wen* (i.e., general questions), forms the basis and the core of the book, embracing the entire realm of medical knowledge. The *Ling shu* (spiritual nucleus) constitutes largely a supplement to the *Su wen*.

During the time of the T'ang Dynasty, probably around A.D. 762, the scholar and minister Wang P'ing added extensive commentaries to the *Nei Ching*, and divided the book into eighty-one chapters. During the Sung Dynasty and later, still more interpretations appeared, but the original commentaries by Wang P'ing were retained in all editions to the present day. Many passages of the *Nei Ching* are practically incomprehensible without these commentaries, since the book's pronouncements are formulated in sparing and terse language and presuppose a sound knowledge of medicine.

The therapies described in the *Nei Ching* are characteristic of Chinese medical thinking. They are almost exclusively directed toward re-establishing disturbed balances, since disrupted harmonies are regarded as the sole cause of disease. In extremely rare instances, surgical operations are recommended, but only as the very last resort, usually for removing malignant tumors.

The entire text of *Nei Ching* is arranged in the form of a dialogue between Huang-ti and his minister Ch'i Po, whose questions and answers touch on almost all fields of medicine. Starting with the concept of *tao* and the cosmological patterns of the universe, the book proceeds to expound in vivid imagery the character of the two primordial forces, *Yin* and *Yang*, and their interrelated performance within nature and within the human being. Then follow descriptions of the organs and explanations of their functions.

A substantial part of the discussion is devoted to the pulse theory, so indispensable to Chinese medical practice. The subtle differentiation between the individual pulse types, as well as the diagnoses derived from the various pulse beats, requires very attentive reading and study. Even then, this is no simple task, although the picturesque descriptions make it somewhat easier.

Very peculiar also are the chapters dealing with the connections between the pulses and the "meridians" (see the sections on pulse theory and acupuncture in the second half

of this book). The minute descriptions of the various types
of fever reveal the enormous knowledge the Chinese possessed on this subject even at such an early time. Especially
valuable in these descriptions are the accounts of the causes
of fever, because they serve to illustrate the thoroughness
with which these ancient physicians observed the course of
fever diseases.

As already mentioned, the second part, *Ling shu*, offers a
supplement and elaborations on the topics contained in
the *Su wen*. Finally, the *Ling shu* treats very exhaustively the
field of acupuncture, which is touched on only briefly in the
first part.

Famous Doctors and Famous Works

HUA T'O, GOD OF SURGERY

An interesting figure is Hua T'o, "God of Surgery," who
lived in the second century A.D. From a mixture of hemp
and wine he developed an excellent anesthetic and was thus
able to perform the most difficult operations completely
painlessly.

Among his many patients was the famous general Kuan
Yün, one of the best-known heroes of Chinese history. With
his height, his large, somewhat protruding eyes, and with his
bristly tiger's beard, he must have been the prototype of the
bold and boisterous warrior. He and his two friends, Liu Pei
and Chang Fei—to whom he was bound by blood-brother-
hood—fought loyally side by side in all battles. Kuan Yün's
courage and daring gained him the admiration of the whole
country. His heroic deeds remained unforgotten among the
people, and in the sixteenth century he was entered into the
circle of the gods. To this day, people make pilgrimages to
the temples erected in his honor as war god and sacrifice
there. Since Kuan Yün during his lifetime, despite his hot
temperament, had always been a chivalrous helper of those
in distress, the ability to heal the sick from the beyond was
eventually ascribed to him.

When this famous Kuan Yün was still fighting on earth,
he appeared one day at Dr. Hua T'o's door in order to have
extracted a poison that an enemy's arrow had shot deeply
into his upper arm. Hua T'o's suggestion of putting him
under narcotics before beginning the operation was laughed
off scornfully by Kuan Yün. Quite unconcerned, he held

out his injured arm to Hua T'o, and while the doctor dug
into the deep wound and cut away the poisoned flesh, Kuan
Yün with the greatest of ease played a round of chess with
one of his friends.

Some time later, Kuan Yün's archenemy, the usurper
Ts'ao Ts'ao, came to Hua T'o and begged him to relieve him
of insufferable headaches. Hua T'o advised him to undergo
an operation on his head; but when the doctor was just
about to perforate the skull, Ts'ao Ts'ao was suddenly
struck with fear and suspicion: Hua T'o might have been
hired by his enemies to murder him cunningly. The physician was thrown into prison and beheaded.

Unfortunately, almost nothing of Hua T'o's extensive
medical writings has been preserved. He is said to have left
instructions before his execution that his entire work should
be destroyed. Another version claims that his wife, knowing
nothing about the inestimable value of the writings, burnt
them in her kitchen stove while her husband lay in prison.

CHANG CHUNG CHING, THE HIPPOCRATES
OF THE EAST

One of the most renowned physicians of the same era was
Chang Chung Ching (c. A.D. 150–200), who is frequently
referred to as the Hippocrates of the East. He owes this
fame largely to his book *Shang Han Lun* (*The Characteristics of Fever Types*), in which he concentrates especially on
diseases of a typhoid nature and recommends a great number of remedies for them. Chang Chung Ching was an extremely prolific writer. Aside from the book mentioned and
the *Chin Chüeh Yau Lüeh* (*Collections of the Golden
Chamber*), he wrote innumerable treatises on medical
themes, including one on women's diseases.

At the time of the Western Chin Dynasty (265–316),
the physician Wang Shu Ho wrote the *Mo Ching*, a treatment of the pulse theory, which made his name immortal.

T'ao Hung Ching and Hsü Chih Ts'ai were two promi-
nent doctors of the Liang period (502–556). T'ao Hung
Ching completed *Pen Ts'ao*, the pharmacological work on
herbs, and Hsü Chih Ts'ai arranged its contents in clear
schematic order.

Although pharmacology was by no means neglected during the Sui Dynasty (589–617), the field of pathology began
to move into the foreground of medical thinking. Under
the auspices of the Imperial Court, Ch'ao Yüan Fang, to-

gether with other physicians, published a voluminous work on the subject of pathology. This book may well be considered one of the best specialized works of its time; many later generations were to extract their medical knowledge from it.

The first dissertation on eye diseases and their therapies (ophthalmology) was the *Yin Hei Ching Wei*; however, the time of its publication can no longer be verified. It has often been regarded as the work of Sun Sze Mo (died A.D. 682), but was probably written much later.

SCHOLARLY DISPUTES AND THE

FORMATION OF SECTS

During the T'ang Dynasty (618–907), important new impulses were felt, not only in art and literature, but also in the field of medicine. All ruling sovereigns of that period furthered the study of medicine and instituted professorial chairs in all specialized medical subjects. It is interesting to note the parallel to our era's trend toward specialization, a development which is often attacked—partly with, but overwhelmingly without, justification.

One of the most remarkable works of this period is the medical encyclopedia of Wang Tao, a gold mine for anyone seeking detailed descriptions of diseases, their symptoms and courses, or old medical prescriptions.

After a rather barren period of five dynasties (907–960), we next encounter at the beginning of the eleventh century a notable "specialist," the pediatrician Ch'ien I. He was seriously ill himself, and is said to have impressed his contemporaries mostly by his extraordinary insights and his capacity for understanding. He developed a number of new drugs for the treatment of children's diseases and removed the panic surrounding many illnesses that had been considered incurable before his time.

The extent to which specialization was carried is apparent in a figure like Pang An Shi. "Professor" Pang, as he would be called today, specialized in the exploration of fevers. During the same period, valuable writings appeared on gynecology and even studies of epidemics and of beriberi, a disease which, as we know today, is caused by a lack of vitamin B.

Feuds among scholars have existed throughout all ages, whether they are disputes on genuine problems or merely bouts of shadow-boxing for the sake of getting one's name known. Often, the less significant the actual results, the louder the battle cries. Old China was no exception. Toward the end of the twelfth century and during the thirteenth century, violent scholarly battles were fought, and fanatical sects began to emerge. One camp would seek to prove, with dogged obstinacy, that heat and cold alone were the causes of all diseases, while the opposing party proclaimed over-abundance and deficiency within the body the only causes. This combatting of sects dragged on through the Yüan Dynasty (1280–1368) and far into the Ming Dynasty (1368–1644).

In the light of such petty quarreling, a figure like Tai Yüan Li (born 1322), who eagerly advocated the ancient theory of *Yin* and *Yang*, must impress us today as extremely "modern."

LI SHIH CHEN AND HIS PHARMACEUTICS

While medical science as such suffered from this discord, the art of pharmacology began to blossom. The most out-standing work of Chinese pharmacology—perhaps of any pharmacology—the *Pen Ts'ao Kang Mu*, was written during that very period. Its author, Li Shih Chen, born at the beginning of the sixteenth century, made it his life's task to prepare this schematic listing of all herbs and drugs. He described every entered item in detail, had illustrations made for each one, added all possible information about its habitat, pointed out specific qualities, usabilities, advantages and disadvantages, and prescribed procedures for extracting the drugs and the dosage for each particular case of illness.

This unique work, which also includes 12,000 recipes for preparing medications, lists not only vegetable sources, but animal substances as well. In its fifty volumes, all species are treated individually, beginning with the elements earth, water, fire and wood. Plants growing from earth, moun-tains, water, rocks, and stones are grouped under separate headings, so are the different kinds of vegetables, fruits, trees, and bushes. Fishes with scales and those without scales, tortoises, crabs, mussels, oysters, and algae are also described individually and in great detail. As part of his research material, Li Shih Chen used the more than forty earlier versions of *Pen Ts'ao*, as well as hundreds of other medical works—an achievement that cannot be valued too highly. An essential feature of his encyclopedia are the directions for the best ways to preserve the drugs.

To describe, even to mention, the endless number of

Chinese medical publications here would be an impossible undertaking. One book, however, deserves to be singled out. Shortly before the end of the Ming Dynasty in 1644, the doctor Wu Yü Hsing issued a fascinating study of the plague.

A significant indication of medical trends during the Ch'ing Dynasty (1644–1911) is the increasing desire to broaden knowledge of the anatomy of the human body. The dissecting of corpses was as illegal then as it had been before, making it impossible for physicians to obtain an exact picture of the organs. Only animals were available for anatomical research. The achievements of a person like Wang Ch'ing Jen, born in 1768, are therefore doubly commendable. With untiring determination, Dr. Wang Ch'ing Jen proceeded to rectify the erroneous conception of human anatomy prevalent at the time. The doctor's special interest was directed toward the exploration of the diaphragm.

Gradually, more and more rumors about the Europeans' superior anatomical knowledge seeped into China; however, it was still some time before contact between European and Chinese medical practices could be established. Even though Europeans were far advanced in anatomical examinations and research apparatus, it was still alien to the Chinese mind to accept diagnoses based on such machinery. To this day, no true marriage of Chinese and Western medical knowledge has been achieved, although more and more Chinese students are studying Western medicine outside their country, and although in the large hospitals in China, patients may choose between Chinese and Western treatment-methods.* The West, in turn, shows a growing interest in Chinese medical methods. The art of acupuncture, especially, has found its followers in Western countries.

DR. LO SHEN MAKES A CALL

When the doctor's bearers had delivered their master's calling-card at the house of the noble Kao, they set down the sedan chair beside the stately portal and waited. Presently the servant, who had been sent by the doorman to take the card to his master, returned. Mr. Kao was ready to receive Dr. Lo Shen! The bearers carried the doctor through two large courts where peach trees stood in full blossom and finally stopped in front of Mr. Kao's drawing

* In Peking, an institute was founded recently for both old Chinese and modern medicine.

room. Dr. Lo Shen slowly emerged from the sedan chair and looked around the hall. With an appreciative glance at the valuable scrolls and the framed written characters hanging on the walls, he entered the room in which Mr. Kao lay.

When the expected visitor had been announced, Mr. Kao had immediately donned his hat and lifted himself from his bed, and was now proceeding to greet Dr. Lo Shen. With a polite gesture of the hand he invited his guest to have a seat. Dr. Lo Shen declined gratefully, as the rules of courtesy dictated, and now on his part, begged Mr. Kao to accommodate himself first. Finally, after several more exchanges of compliments and bows, both gentlemen sat down.

A servant appeared with a tray on which were two bowls and a small pot of tea. Mr. Kao took one bowl gracefully in both hands and presented it to Dr. Lo Shen, whereupon the latter offered a bowl to his host. "I have heard much of your great abilities and your art, my lord," began the doctor, opening the conversation as protocol ruled the guest should do. "May I ask your age?"

"I am a completely incapable person and have so far spent fifty-three useless years," replied Mr. Kao. "Of your fame and your wisdom, dear doctor, I have known for a long time."

"My knowledge, alas, is only very slight," Dr. Lo Shen protested modestly. In properly chosen words he now congratulated Mr. Kao on his three gifted sons, whereupon Mr. Kao, in turn, rejected this praise modestly and declared that his sons were, alas, completely untalented and worthless human beings.

During this conversation, Dr. Lo Shen did not fail to study very closely Mr. Kao's complexion. He immediately detected that the inner corners of his host's eyes had a yellowish color, a favorable sign for his general disposition. After a further test of courteous exchanges, Mr. Kao arrived at the real reason for asking the doctor to his house.

"For several days now I have felt rather tired and have had no appetite." It did not escape the doctor that Mr. Kao's voice was slightly husky. He now turned to his host and asked if he might see his tongue. When he had studied it for a while and drawn his conclusions from its appearance, he then asked Mr. Kao to let him feel his pulse. Mr. Kao pushed back the long sleeve of his black, fur-lined silk robe and stretched out his arm to the doctor. "May I ask you to tell me what is wrong?" he inquired of Lo Shen. The doctor took the left wrist of the patient and pressed his ring finger on the spot where the palm is separated from the lower arm, placing middle and index fingers right next to it. Now, for a half-hour or more, he examined each one of the three pulses individually, using light, medium, and then firm pressure, at the same time counting the patient's intakes of breath. After that, he took Mr. Kao's right wrist with his right hand, placed his index finger on the spot where palm and lower arm meet, and placed middle and ring finger close to it. His thumb rested on the ball of the patient's hand. Again, one half-hour or more passed.

"Aside from the heart pulse—which seems a trifle weak and, unfortunately, does not feel like a string of pearls—the pulses are rather reassuring," began Dr. Lo Shen. "A very favorable symptom is the good condition of the liver pulse, which, as you know, corresponds to the present season of spring. One might compare it to a gently stretched lute-string. When you urinate," asked the doctor, "do you have a strong headache?"

"I would not go so far as to say that." replied Mr. Kao; "sometimes, it is true, there is a kind of numbness, but it cannot really be called a headache."

Dr. Lo Shen nodded. "I thought so. If I may be so bold as to announce freely my opinion, I would like to state that yours is a case of the hundred combinations disease, which was probably caused by a cold that was overlooked."

"I still have shivers now and then," agreed the patient. "Although we are having such mild days, I sometimes cannot fight this feeling of chill."

"That is very characteristic of the illness," remarked Dr. Lo Shen, "and so are the paleness in your face and the tenseness of the root of your tongue. Still, it is a good sign that you have no headache when you urinate, for then you may recover in twenty days. Do not worry yourself when you feel low and fatigued: those are the accompanying symptoms of the illness that, unfortunately, you have to bear with. Most likely, you will also get a slight cough."

"How shall I take care of the illness?"

"I would like to ask you to rest as much as possible and not to strain your eyes. Every kind of exertion will affect your heart, which is at present somewhat weakened. A light toning with acupuncture should bring you relief very soon, and, if you permit, I should like to perform it this very moment."

When Dr. Lo Shen had finished the acupuncture, he gave Mr. Kao some advice on his diet and prescribed for him a drug to strengthen the heart. Then he took his leave and promised to come back after a few days.

At all times in history, there have been doctors who would risk their lives for the sick. Nor were the rulers a rarity who, dissatisfied with their doctors' services, would make them suffer cruelly. The following legend from the *Lü Shih Ch'un Ch'iu* may illustrate how beloved the theme of a physician's ethics was even then.

DR. WEN CHI SACRIFICES HIS LIFE

The ministers of Chi were distraught. For weeks now the King had not shown the slightest interest in the affairs of the State and had been oblivious of everything that went on around him. He who had always been energetic and active lay in bed in complete apathy, moaning at intervals in his deep melancholia. Every bit of food that he had swallowed during the past weeks had been vomited immediately. While his ministers stood around his bed and recited their reports, the King would stare into space, unmoved. Finally, the King's son decided to send for the renowned doctor Wen Chi.

Wen Chi obeyed the call and examined the King thoroughly. He examined each of the pulses separately, observed the tongue and the face color for a long time, and listened attentively to the moaning voice of the patient. Then he left the King's bedchamber and announced that he would return the next day at the same hour.

"His Excellency's condition is very serious," he said to the Prince before leaving. "His emotional depression must be lifted from him at once, otherwise he is lost. I fear, alas, that if I save him, it will cost me my own life."

When the Prince asked what he meant by that remark, Wen Chi replied thoughtfully: "Only if I succeed in throwing him into a terrible fury, only then can he recover. But if I do that, he will have me executed."

The Prince implored the doctor to try everything in his power to keep the King alive and promised him that he should not have to fear for his own life. The Prince as well as the Queen would take care that no harm should befall him. On the next day at the prescribed hour, the King was waiting for the visit of the doctor. But hour after hour passed, and Wen Chi did not appear. Neither did a servant appear to explain the doctor's tardiness. Such rudeness was noticeable even to the King in his prostrate condition, and he became restless and nervous. And when during the following day the King had to wait again in vain for Wen Chi, a dreadful anger began to well up inside him.

Finally, after four days had elapsed, Dr. Wen Chi suddenly appeared before the King. Without taking off his shoes, he strode up to the King's bedside and snapped a few questions at him, all the while scraping his dirty shoes over the King's fine silk robes. To make matters worse, he now proceeded to direct a stream of insults and abuse at the patient. At last, the King could no longer contain himself. Trembling with fury, he jumped up from his bed and ordered his ministers to grab the doctor and punish him for his outrageous behavior by throwing him into a kettle of boiling oil.

No sooner had the King shouted these words than he felt himself completely refreshed, demanded a ten-course dinner, and was relieved of all his ailments.

Prince and Queen were horror-struck when they heard what the King had done and begged him to retract the punishment. But there was no trace of the earlier apathy left now in the King's mind, and he insisted on the immediate execution of his command. The hangmen seized Dr. Wen Chi and threw him into the sizzling oil. For three days and nights he suffered excruciating tortures without being released by death.

"You must close the kettle with a lid; only then will my life be extinguished," Wen Chi lectured the hangmen.

His words were reported to the King, who ordered the kettle to be covered with a lid. And Wen Chi could finally give up his life.

PHYSICIAN—A DANGEROUS PROFESSION

Although most rulers were well disposed toward their healers, doctors had to live in constant fear of losing such benevolence should they ever fail in their treatments. This arbitrary behavior is best documented by Emperor I Tsung, who reigned from A.D. 860 to 874. His daughter, whom he loved above all else, fell severely ill and the Emperor called to his court one doctor after another from all corners of the empire. But none was able to save her. Embittered, the Emperor had them all executed. There were more than twenty of them.

TSANG KUNG AND HIS COURAGEOUS DAUGHTER

Dr. Chun Yü I, who was born in 207 B.C. and later came to be known by the name Tsang Kung, was a diagnostician of the highest repute. The greatest honors were bestowed on him by the Imperial Court. However, he was also a rather peculiar and obstinate person and refused repeatedly to visit certain sick people. Thus he eventually forfeited the favor of the Emperor and was sentenced to have his limbs cut off. One of his five daughters—his marriage had not been blessed with a single son—accompanied him to Chang An. There she submitted a petition to the Emperor, asking him to pardon her father and to take her instead into bondage as a slave. Emperor Wen Ti was so moved by the girl's courage and her filial devotion that he remitted her father's punishment and later even issued an edict abolishing punishment by mutilation.

CHUNG K'UEI, THE EXORCISER

Emperor Hsüan of the T'ang Dynasty was tossing on his bed in feverish dreams. A malevolent demon had wormed his way into the palace, mocking the sick Emperor, who was helplessly delivered to the demon's wiles. Suddenly one day, the giant figure of a man wearing high boots and a hat punctured with holes appeared in the Emperor's bedchamber. He threw himself on the monster, battered him down with a heavy club, and tore out one of the monster's eyes and swallowed it.

"Who are you?" gasped the Emperor.

"I am Dr. Chung K'uei," came the reply. "More than a hundred years ago, I reported for the State medical examination, but the jury of professors very unjustly failed me. I could not live on with such shame and took my own life in front of Emperor Kao Tsu's palace. The Emperor, who received word of my suicide, investigated the matter and then had me buried with high honors in order to rehabilitate my name. I therefore vowed never to forget this kindness of the Imperial House and to come to the rescue of all emperors who are being molested by demons."

The Emperor awakened and found that the fever had left him. The next day he sent for the famous artist Wu Tao Tze and described the apparition to him. Wu Tao Tze painted a picture of Chung K'uei based on the Emperor's tale, which, as the ruler claimed, portrayed exactly the features of his rescuer. Chung K'uei has since then been worshiped as a god and is asked for help especially against persecution by evil spirits and at the outbreak of epidemics.

THE PILL OF IMMORTALITY

A man had brought a small pill to the King of Ch'u—a pill of immortality. When the court attendant carried the pill into the reception hall, an officer intercepted him and asked if the little round object could really be eaten.

"Certainly," answered the attendant, whereupon the officer grabbed the pill from the tray and swallowed it.

The King, furious over such an iniquitous deed, ordered that the officer be executed.

As his last wish, the officer asked to have the following message sent to the King: "It was said that the pill was an immortality pill. If I should be killed now, it would be a sign that the pill is worthless, and His Royal Highness will have made a fool of himself in the eyes of the people."

When the King heard the message, he thought it wiser to revoke the officer's death sentence.

The wish to prolong life or to defeat death altogether with the help of a drug has occupied the minds of men since time immemorial. Some doctors have dedicated their whole lives to such researches. A number of Taoists, so legend tells us, succeeded in finding answers to the eternal quest.

CHANG TAO LIN, THE HIGH PRIEST

OF THE TAOISTS

Eminent among the physicians who subscribed whole-heartedly to Taoistic beliefs was the figure of Dr. Chang Tao Lin, born A.D. 34. He is said to have read the most difficult philosophical texts at the age of seven and to have astounded his elders with his extraordinary intelligence. Although he was later offered many high positions at the Royal Court, he declined all such honors. He preferred to live as a hermit, in order to devote himself entirely to his Taoist meditations and alchemistic studies. The Chinese call him "High Priest of the Taoists." Legend has woven much supernatural ornamentation into his life and work. From the philosopher Lao-tzu he is said to have received, in mysterious manner, a text describing a life-prolonging elixir. The study of this text enabled him to develop his magical talents so far that his spiritual self could abandon his body whenever he wished and could fly to far distances. He is also reported to have halted thunderstorms and to have subjugated demons to his will. At the age of 123 years, so legend has it, he ascended into the heavens, accompanied by his two favorite disciples.

Chang Tao Lin wrote treatises on the expelling of diseases by exorcism. In the course of this, he created innumerable adjuration formulas and talismans which are used in China at the present day. There is hardly a disease for which he did not write a special incantation.

KINGS OF TAOIST MEDICINE

Equally famous is the Taoist scholar Ko Hung, who was born around the middle of the third century. His main interests, too, were the study of alchemy and the search for drugs that would ensure immortality. The works he left behind, however, not only treat of supernatural subjects, but also contain practical instructions on the mixing of medications for acute illnesses. His collection of medical prescriptions, published under the pseudonym Pao Pu Tze, is a first-class achievement.

Another Taoist physician and scholar, Sun Sze Mo (died A.D. 682), gained eternal fame through one of his compilations of prescriptions. This work, the *Chien Chin Yao Fang* (*The Thousand Golden Prescriptions*), as well as the sequel to it, the *Chien Chin I Fang* (*Another Thousand Golden Prescriptions*), won him the highest esteem of the reigning emperor, Tai Tsung, and the epithet Yao Wang (King of Medicine). His research studies on the different types of fever are recognized even today. Beyond that, he is still remembered during the fifth month of the Chinese year, the "month of epidemics," when crowds of worshipers flock to his temples to seek his support and to give thanks.

FEMALE PHYSICIANS, MIDWIVES,

AND FEMALE SHAMANS

Doctors who were summoned to the palace to treat a female member of the emperor's household were confronted with particular difficulties. The rules of etiquette were extremely strict in forbidding any direct contact with a woman patient. To make a pulse diagnosis possible under such conditions, the doctor had a ribbon wrapped around the patient's wrist, with one end left dangling. The doctor would then try to feel the pulse from that end of the bandage.

Very little is known about the activities of female doctors, although it is apparent from history that many women possessed considerable medical talents. Historical chronicles report of a female who let herself be bribed into mixing poison into the meals of the wife of Emperor Hsüan Ti (73–48 B.C.). The lady was to be murdered so that the daughter of a general might become empress after the former's death.

Legend further tells how Hsi Wang Mu (Mother of the West) very skillfully removed a boil from the leg of a man who was later to become one of the "eight immortals." In fact, it was through her that he acquired the magic of staying immortal.

Finally, mention must be made of the female shamans. Possessing the fundamental gifts of prophetesses, they were able to dance themselves into trances and, in a state of ecstasy, exert lasting influence upon their fellow beings. But they were generally feared, because they were wild, like furies, in their frenzy. Around 500 B.C., a female shaman appears in the writings of the philosopher Lieh Tze: "She knew all about the death of a person, and all about his birth. Her pronouncements fell upon humankind like the words of gods. Wherever she appeared, men, women, and children would hide their faces or flee from her path."

III

MEDICINAL HERBS,

DRUGS, AND LOVE-MEDICINES

The little town of Kun Hsien was hustling and bustling with excitement, for today was the fifth day of the fifth month, the day on which precautionary measures had to be taken against illnesses and against the influence of evil spirits.

Immediately upon getting up in the morning, Mrs. Chang had carried around her votive offerings—rice and meat to Yao Wang, the King of Medicine, and assorted tidbits of food to T'ou Chen Niang Niang, the Goddess of the Pox. Nor had she forgotten to offer lotus-flower seeds and a small bowl of tea to the goddess Kuan Yin. Her favors had to be secured for the forthcoming birth of a grandchild. Mrs. Chang's daughter-in-law was already in her seventh month of pregnancy, and the grace of Kuan Yin would make delivery easier and would, above all, ensure that the baby was a boy. Still, to be absolutely certain, Mrs. Chang had already picked the motherwort (*Leonurus sibiricus*), in order to to have it ready when the time came.

"I do hope you have not allowed yourselves any carelessness this time, as you did last year," she said as she turned to her sons, "for it was your fault, surely, that your little sister Mei Hua died. Never before had the one-hundred-herb medicine failed to work."

The sons were silent. Each one asked himself if it had not been he who had made the fatal mistake. Mei Hua's death had been a hard blow for all of them. She was only a girl, it was true, yet their parents had spared no effort to save her life. But that even the one-hundred-herb medicine had failed was serious reason for worry. "In the very early morning hours, you must go exactly one hundred steps into the meadow and, without looking east or west, you must pick one hundred grasses," demanded the centuries-old instruction. "If the number of steps or the number of grasses is not exactly one hundred, or if one single ray of sunshine touches

41

the grasses, the medicine loses its power." Who could tell now which of them had counted wrong last year?

"Do not worry yourself, Mother," the eldest son tried to comfort Mrs. Chang, "this year we certainly did not make any mistakes. Each of us put his one hundred herbs into the big kettle directly after sunrise. They have now been cooking for almost four hours. Soon we shall be able to strain the brew and pour it into bottles."

"You did not, I hope, use a metal pot?" asked Mrs. Chang anxiously.

"But Mother, how can you even imagine such a thing!" cried the sons, utterly shocked.

Somewhat reassured, the mother sat down at the table and put a thimbleful of mugwort (*Artemisia vulgaris*—absinthe) into the tiny bag of red silk that she had sewn for her four-year-old daughter, Mei Ling, and had embroidered with the emblems of long life. When the girl wore the mugwort bag on a string around her neck, no evil spirits could overpower her. As an added protection, the mother had stitched a small bell with a clear-ringing sound onto her daughter's cap.

Now Mrs. Chang had to check her stock of medicines. Was the dried ginger preserved well? Were there still enough dates, orange rinds, and peach seeds in the house? The supply of ginseng extract was frighteningly low and had to be replenished. Plasters, too, were missing, and she had to buy resin to prepare new ones.

Finally, when she had fumigated all the rooms of the house with strong-smelling herbs to impede the entry of evil spirits, she could rest assured that she had taken all necessary precautions to extinguish quickly any outbreak of illness.

Medicinal Herbs in Old China

The position of curative herbs in medicine has been a constant cause for argument between academic science on one side and practical folk-experience on the other. The fruitless battles are now gradually subsiding. Even in orthodox strongholds of medicine, a doctor appears now and then who will risk his reputation and try again a forgotten little herb. The fact that certain businessmen—more or less dishonorable—try to turn many a discovery, or rediscovery, into a sensational "remedy for all ills" does not reduce the genuine medicinal value of some herbs.

Quack practices must have existed even in the China of

old, for the number of diseases that are supposedly cured with one or another popular herb is legion. The ginseng, for instance, which is becoming popular again in Europe, is recommended for the following diseases—among others:

Anemia	Headaches
Asthma	Heart failure
Chest and stomach aches	Impotence
Colds and fever	Indigestion
Colics	Insomnia
Complications after difficult childbirth	Lack of appetite
Depression	Menstrual disorders
Dizzy spells	Nausea
Dropsy	Nervous disorders
Excessive thirst	Old-age weakness
Exhaustion	Rheumatism
Eye weakness	Vascular cramps

With the help of the existing textbooks, this list may be extended or adjusted at random.

Obviously, the Chinese had the same experience as Europeans and perhaps all people who seize upon remedies without proper testing methods: they fell victim to superstition. The *signatura rerum*, which appears in European herb-therapies of the past, is a perfect example: a plant is effective against diseases of that organ whose shape it resembles. The stoneweed, with its small, hard and round nutlets, produces a tea against kidney stones; the crowfoot species *Anemone hepatica*, with its leaves shaped like livers, is effective against liver ailments, and so forth.

The Chinese developed this still further. When the mere name of the plant resembled that of the disease, the plant was considered a sympathetic remedy. Moreover, all plants whose names sounded like good-luck words were endowed with appropriate therapeutic qualities.

Superstition also overwhelmed ideas that may have held some basic truth; for example, the recognition that the gathering season of a herb was important to its effect. The ghost hours, the full moon, and all the paraphernalia of magicians of yore were called in to steep everything in an aura of mystery. Bringing it down to a realistic level can be rewarding; one may discover that certain plants do, indeed, retain their active ingredients only as long as the dew has not dried on their leaves.

GINSENG—THE MAN-SHAPED ROOT

The mandrake has always held a special charm for the peoples of Europe. With the slightest bit of imagination, this root, with its fleshy arms and knuckles, may be turned into a tiny human creature.

So, too, can the homely little ginseng root lure one into intriguing fantasies. Its branches become arms and legs, while a knotty bulb here and a blotchy spot there emerge as a human face.

Just as the mandrake root must be harvested at a prescribed hour and by a definite ritual, so does Chinese ritual require the ginseng root to be dug out only at midnight of a full moon, if it is to be of any worth.

Now, even as in the past, the growing and selling of the man-shaped root is a profitable business. At various times in its history, it has been worth its weight in silver, or five times its weight in gold. During the reign of Tao Kuang (1821–1851), people were so greedy for ginseng that a special decree was issued to protect the plant from extinction (consider the fate of the gentian and arnica in the West!).

But what does this wonder-root that the Chinese call *Jen shen* really contain and when is it effective? A chemical examination reveals the following constituents in the *Panax ginseng* and its related species, *Panax quinquefolius* (the American ginseng): resin, a saponin, starch, tannin, aromatic bitters, volatile oils, and traces of panacin. It is probably the latter to which many of the root's healing powers may be ascribed. Ginseng tastes bitter at first, then turns sweet because of its starch content.

It is assumed that the ginseng's therapeutic value is due to its non-specific action. However, research on this subject has by no means been exhausted. So far, there is no agreement at all on the true value of the root. It can be said with certainty, though, that here and there it is being used with surprising results. In some persons it is reported to have increased the sexual powers. Even if these reports are honest, however, they alone do not prove that the heightened potency is really caused by the ginseng; for, surely, the people who take an aphrodisiac are merely those who have already an urgent drive toward lovemaking. It remains to be clarified how much of it is one's own eagerness, imagination, and faith in the powers of the root, and how much of it is due to actual chemical action. Still, it would be folly to brush aside as mere imagination all remedial properties of this or any herb that has maintained its reputation through centuries and millennia.

Recipes for the Preparation of Herb Medicines, and Their Application

Without doubt, man owes the discovery of medicinal plants to the same instinct that can be observed to a certain extent in animals. They, too, use particular plants only in times of particular illnesses, while at other times they leave the same plant untouched, or avoid it deliberately.

When comparing the medicinal plants known to the Chinese with the herbals of other peoples, the conformity between them is so striking that one might suspect their authors to have copied from one another. Not only do the plants' properties coincide, but often also the preparation procedures and the suggested uses. Orange peel appears almost without exception as a component of sedatives; the willow is invariably used for rheumatism. (The willow, *salix*, contains salicylic acid, hence its working mechanism is the same as that of aspirin. Salicylamides are still used as remedies for acute rheumatism, despite modern cortisone and ACTH—Adreno-Cortico-Trophic Hormone of the pituitary gland.)

MAJOR TYPES OF MEDICAL PRESCRIPTIONS

Ta-fang: Large prescriptions with many ingredients.
Hsiao-fang: Small prescriptions with few ingredients.
Huan-fang: Slow prescriptions for tonics with reviving qualities.
Ch'i-fang: Prescriptions with an odd number of ingredients.
Wu-fang: Prescriptions with an even number of ingredients.

The Main Rules for Preparing Prescriptions

Different diseases require differently prepared medications.

Liquid medications serve to cleanse the intestines, to stimulate the blood circulation and to restore the balance between *Yin* and *Yang*.

Pills are used for alleviating stagnations and congestions and for removing cold and wind from the body.

Powders are to be taken for stomach and intestinal afflictions.

Illnesses caused by action of cold upon the body should be subdued with hot medicines; while cold medications should be administered for illnesses caused by heat.

Medicines for ailments above the chest should be taken after meals.

Medicines for ailments below the heart and stomach should be taken before meals.

Medicines for sickness in the four limbs should be taken early in the morning on an empty stomach.

For afflictions of bones and marrow: in the evening after a meal.

Soups, brews, and other liquid medications are best for severe diseases, medications in pill form are best for diseases that develop gradually, and medicines in powder form are to be used for suddenly erupting diseases.

Herbs must not be cooked in utensils made of metal; the most satisfactory are earthenware containers. For cutting the herbs, no metal knives may be used; use cutting tools of bamboo or a similar material. Likewise, mortars in which herbs are ground must not be of metal.

CHINESE WEIGHTS AND MEASURES

1 *chin* =	16 *liang* =	576.00 grams
1 *liang* =	10 *chien* =	36.00 grams
1 *chien* =	10 *fen* =	3.60 grams
1 *fen* =	10 *li* =	0.36 grams
1 *li* =		0.036 grams
1 *shu* =		1.56 grams
1 *chu* =	100 millet seeds	
1 *tou* =	10 *sheng* =	˙10.35 liters
1 *sheng* =	10 *ho* =	1.035 liters
1 *ho* =		0.1035 liter
1 *chang* =	10 *ch'ih* =	approximately 3.048 meters
1 *ch'ih* =	10 *ts'un* =	approximately 0.3048 meters
1 *ts'un* =	10 *fen* =	approximately 2.54 centimeters
1 *fen* =		approximately 0.254 centimeters

Ginseng and Other Prescriptions

Basic Rule: Ginseng must not be prepared in metal vessels. For storing, only crockery should be used. In exceptional cases it may be left in silver containers.

Ginseng essence: Cook ginseng in water until only a sediment remains; this should be pressed into a crock and stored.

To stimulate digestion: Rub ginseng to powder and dissolve it in the white of an egg; mixture must be taken three times a day.

To strengthen the heart and to avert depression: Blend one *liang* of pulverized ginseng with ten *liang* of lard and dissolve this mixture in good wine, twice a day a small bowl of this.

As a sedative: Prepare a light broth of ginseng and bamboo leaves.

As a restorative for frail children: Give a dash of raw, minced ginseng several times a day.

To stimulate blood circulation: One small bowlful of ginseng potion mixed with honey and *Cinnamomum cassia* (cinnamon); to be drunk once a day.

For faintness after childbirth: Administer a strong brew of ginseng several times a day.

For insomnia: An extract made of equal parts of chopped ginseng and dried orange peel, fortified with honey; to be swallowed before going to bed.

For stiffness in the joints: Prepare an extract of two parts ginseng and one part *Eucommia ulmoides* (rubber tree); to be taken on an empty stomach.

To settle the stomach: Prepare a brew of one part *Astragalus hoantschy* (vetch species) and two parts ginseng; to be sipped before meals.

Against fever: Cook one *liang* of ginseng in two cups of water; boil this down to half the quantity; add a shot of pure spring or well water; will induce perspiration immediately.

To remove the consequences of sexual excesses: Cook green ginger together with orange peel and stir into ginseng essence.

For general failing, especially in old people: Mix raw ginger juice with honey and ginseng and boil this down until it just covers the bottom of the pot; cut nut-sized lumps from it, dissolve them in hot water in which rice has been cooked, and feed them to the patient.

For nausea, urinary difficulties, short-windedness, headache, and swollen eyes:

Paeonia albiflora	3 *liang*
Cinnamomum cassia	3 *liang* (without skin)
Glycyrrhiza glabra	3 *liang* (raw)
Zyziphus vulgaris	12 pieces

For colds, headaches, and prolonged constipation:

Cinnamomum cassia	4 *liang* (without skin)
Aconitum fischeri	3 pieces
Zingiber officinale	3 *liang* (raw)
Zyziphus vulgaris	12 pieces

Cook in 6 *sheng* of water; boil it down to 4 *sheng*.

For outer heat and inner coldness, dry palate, cold hands and feet, limpness of body (this medication is known as the white-tiger potion and may also be administered without *Panax ginseng;* it produces sweat and quenches thirst):

Anemarrhena asphodeloides	6 *liang*
Gypsum	1 *chin* (pounded to powder)
Glycyrrhiza glabra	2 *liang*
Oryza sativa	6 *ho*
Panax ginseng	3 *liang*

For injury of the kidneys through cold and dampness, when the body is heavy and the waist is cold and bloated as though one were sitting in water. When the belly, too, is heavy as though 5,000 gold pieces were stored in it, and the lower warmer is so full of sweat that it drenches the clothing:

Glycyrrhiza glabra	2 *liang*
Zingiber officinale	2 *liang*
Heterosmilax	4 *liang*
Atractylis ovata, white	2 *liang*

Cook in 5 *sheng* of water; boil it down to 2 *sheng;* take it three times a day.

As a restorative:

Panax ginseng	3 *liang*
Zingiber officinale	3 *liang*
Atractylis ovata, white	3 *liang*

Cook in 8 *sheng* of water and boil it down to 5 *sheng;* drink 1 *sheng* lukewarm three times a day.

A B C of Chinese Medicinal Plants

In the following compendium of medicinal plants, the Chinese, Latin, and, where one exists, English name is given for each herb. Wherever the authors have thought it of interest, they have added information on further uses, compiled from herbals and dispensatories:

*Aconitum fischeri—Fu-tze—*Azure Monkshood, or Wolfsbane
A very popular medication, also used as a subsidiary ingredient in other medicines. It is said to be effective against smallpox, diarrhea, fever, colds, and coughs.

*Aconitum uncinatum—Ts'ao wu t'ou—*Clambering Monkshood
The pulverized root is mixed with the white of a raw egg and applied to swellings and bruises.

Almost all types of monkshood, or wolfsbane, contain rather large quantities of aconite, a substance so active and so exceedingly poisonous that for the Romans the word *aconitum* meant poison. Aconite affects the cardiac and respiratory functions and reduces fever. This effect is ascribed to the poison's influence on the autonomic nervous system; for aconite works as an irritant on the "cooling center," i.e., the counter pole to the fever center in the body.

The instruction to administer the pulverized root, mixed with egg white, to swellings and bruises may also have a deeper significance, since aconite can also act as a local pain-reliever. As with all such poisons, there is of course only a hair's breadth between the beneficial and the deadly dosage.

*Acorus calamus—Ch'ang p'u—*Sweet Flag
Strengthening and life-prolonging herb.
The root of the calamus, which is the part used, undoubtedly stimulates the appetite through its content of volatile oils (asarin, calamus camphor, bitters, tannin, etc.) and is also recommended as a medication for inflammation of the gastric membrane, and for colic. In Arabia and Iran it is reputed to intensify sexual potency.

*Adenophora polymorpha—Sha shen—*Fickle Ladybell
Used in cases of pulmonary diseases.

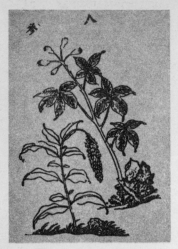

Fig. 2. *Panax ginseng*
Ginseng, the Man-shaped
Root.

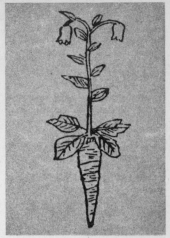

Fig. 3. *Adenophora poly-
morpha* Fickle Ladybell.

Fig. 4. *Asarum sieboldi*
Species of Wild Ginger.

Fig. 5. *Atractylis ovata.*

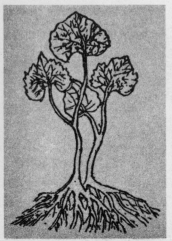

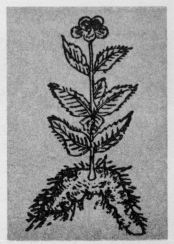

Aesculus chinensis—T'ien shih li—Chinese Horse-Chestnut
Widely used remedy for rheumatism.

Aloe vulgaris L.—Lu hui—Mediterranean Aloe
Well-known purgative of age-old repute. Not recommended for pregnant women.

Amomum cardamomum—Pai t'ou k'ou—Cardamom (of the ginger family)
Effective remedy for spells of weakness and fever.
Cardamomi fructus, the fruits of various ginger plants, are listed in European and American pharmacopoeias as stomachics and aromatics. They are also used as medicine in India, besides being a flavoring agent in curry.

Anemarrhena asphodeloides—Chih mu
A popular remedy for head colds accompanied by fever.

Angelica polymorpha—Tang kuei—species of Angelica
Good blood-cleanser; said to remove hemorrhoids and menstrual disorders; dilates the blood vessels and draws pus in boils.
All species of angelica contain a number of volatile oils that affect the heart, the blood circulation, and the respiration, and contain some antispasmodic components. The varied use of the herb is therefore quite plausible.

Arctium lappa—Niu p'ang tze—Great Burdock
Promotes bowel movement and discharge of urine. Disperses swellings and ulcers and heals skin rashes.
The root and leaves of the burdock were regarded as medicinal in former times and are today again recommended by some European schools of medicine (including homeopathy) for the treatment of excessive phlegm in air ducts and for skin diseases.

Areca catechu—Ping lang—Betelnut Palm
Used for constipation and for curing serious swellings.

Artemisia capillaris—Yin ch'en—species of Wormwood
Diaphoretic; used to dispel heat from the lungs and for headaches, vertigo, and jaundice.

Artemisia dracunculus—Ch'ing hao—Tarragon
Cures fever, dysentery, and malignant ulcers.

*Artemisia vulgaris—Ai yen—*Mugwort Wormwood

This common mugwort is made into the combustible cones used in moxa cautery. Said to be effective in severe diarrhea and menstrual disturbances.

Artemisia vulgaris has been known in the West also as a medicinal herb. Medical science has banished it from the dispensary, but perhaps unjustly so, since only recently a cholagogic (agent promoting the flow of bile) was discovered in the herb. In folk medicine and in homeopathy it still finds its uses. Its relative, *Artemisia absinthium*, is sometimes abused by employing it to induce abortions. It contains thujone (the strong poison inherent in the occidental white cedar, *Thuya occidentalis*), which may cause severe damage when taken in large, sometimes even in moderate, doses. The sale of absinthe (the liquor) is prohibited in many countries because of the danger of addiction. The spicy absinthe-vermouth contains virtually none of the volatile, poisonous oils, but retains the aromatic bitters absinthin, which stimulate the appetite and restore strength.

*Asarum sieboldi—Hsi hsin—*species of Wild Ginger

Effective for blocked-up noses and head colds. Used as a diaphoretic and also a good remedy for eyes watering in sharp wind, as well as for hearing defects.

Asarum camphor (asarone, or asarin) belongs among the ancient medicines. Its root was used as an emetic and diuretic, but has such strong side effects that it was eventually discarded from the field of pharmacology.

*Asparagus lucidus—T'ien men tung—*Shiny Asparagus

Softens dry coughs, removes heat and pains in the feet, cures swellings and ulcers, and strengthens the lungs.

Asparagus used to be prescribed as a diuretic.

*Astragalus hoantschy—Huang ch'i—*species of Loco Weed (Milk Vetch, Poison Vetch)

Can induce perspiration as well as dispel it; when eaten in cooked form, the plant is blood-forming and drains pus from boils; it fortifies the three "warmers," the spleen, and the stomach.

Atractylis ovata—P'ai chu

Works as a tonic, removes constipation, blood congestion, dropsy, and jaundice, and is a good remedy for all cases where the symptoms indicate a malfunction of the spleen.

*Bambusa—Chu hsun—*Bamboo

The bran of bamboo sprouts (there are about fifty species of bamboo in China) is said to be effective in cases of nausea. Roasted bamboo sprouts are a culinary delight and are served as a side dish to meat courses in Chinese restaurants all over the world.

*Brunella vulgaris—Hsia ku ts'ao—*Common Selfheal (Prunella)

Cures colds; removes scrofulous swellings; used to allay pains in the eyes.

*Bupleurum falcatum—Ch'ail hu—*species of Thoroughwax (with sickle-shaped leaves)

Pulls fresh aura into upper part of body; cures head colds, fever, nausea, anxieties, dizzy spells, eye weakness, and pains in chest and head; strengthens the limbs; especially recommended for toning up leg muscles.

Cassia angustifolia (various species)*—Fan hsieh yeh—*Senna

Popular cathartic.

The leaves of the dried senna are utilized as a laxative wherever they grow naturally or are cultivated. They contain emodin, which is also a constituent of such plants as rhubarb, buckthorn, and castor bean.

*Chenopodium ambrosioides L.—T'u ching chieh—*Wormseed Goosefoot (Mexican Tea)

Diaphoretic; strengthens eyes and circulation; cures hemoptysis (blood-coughing), gonorrhea, dysentery; neutralizes poisons in the body and expels intestinal worms.

*Cimicifuga foetida—Sheng ma—*Skunk Bugbane

Neutralizes poisons; relieves headaches.

*Cinnamomum cassia—Kuei—*Cassiabark Tree (Cinnamon)

Regulates stomach and liver temperatures; acts as a carminative and improves the appetite; also widely used in the preparation of incense.

*Clematis recta L.—Mu t'ung—*Ground Clematis (related to Virgin's Bower)

Alleviates heat in the thorax; cleanses the urine; effective against dropsy, deafness, disturbed vision, sore throats, dry

palate, and dry tongue (but not to be taken when perspiration is present).

This species of clematis—formerly medicinally used under the name Flame of Jupiter—is recommended in old and new herbals for diseases of the male genitals, gonorrhea and its complications, prostatomegaly (enlargement of the prostate gland), and even for "a propensity to cancer." Its main active ingredient is amonin, a camphor that is also present in *Anemone pulsatilla.*

Cnicus sinensis L.—Ta hsiao chi—species of Blessed Thistle (Safflower)
Mobilizes the Ch'i *in the body; removes congestions in the blood (hyperemia) and malignant intestinal tumors.*

The *Cnicus benedictus,* native to southern Europe and the Near East, is utilized as a bitters, and acts as an emetic in larger doses. The tannin and mucilage components of the herb may explain its usage for intestinal complaints.

Cocculus thunbergii D. D.—Mu fang chi—species of Snailseed
Mu fang chi achieves good results in asthma, dropsy, swellings, and ulcers; cleanses the blood.

*Coix lacryma jobi L.—I I—*Job's Tears
Widely used diuretic and purgative; also employed in the treatment of rheumatism.

*Coptis sinensis—Huang lien—*Chinese species of Goldthread
The dried root serves well in cases of diarrhea, fever, and swellings in the face.

*Cucumus citrullus—Hsi kua—*species of Melon
This watermelon quenches thirst and soothes inflamed throats.

Watermelons were one of the main causes of the spread of typhus epidemics in China. A European bacteriologist summoned to China for help demanded that an edict be issued forbidding the sale of sliced or cut watermelons. Beyond that, people learned to get into the habit of pouring scalding water over the melons before eating them. By these simple measures, it was possible to conquer several epidemics.

*Curcuma longa—Chiang huang—*Curcuma Root (Turmeric)
Heals wounds and other injuries; relieves pains in the

limbs; dissolves blood congestions; restorative effect after loss of blood at birth of child.

*Curcuma longa var. macrophylla—Yü chin—*Wild Curcuma Root (Bloodroot)
Dissolves stagnations that hinder the forming of new blood; cures cases of bloody sputum and bloody urine; alleviates menstrual complaints, and is generally used as a tonic and stimulant.

The rootstock is sometimes used by scientific medicine in the treatment of functional disorders of the gall bladder and biliary ducts. No satisfying research results exist, however, on the plant's virtues as claimed by the Chinese.

*Cyrtomium fortunei I. Sm.—Shih chung—*species of the Fern family
Solidifies the bones; destroys parasites in the body.

*Daphne genkwa—Yüan hua—*Lilac Daphne (related to Mezereum and Laurel)
Diuretic; effective against fever, respiratory difficulties, and coughing.

The mezereum herbs—formerly medicinally used—contain as their main active ingredient mezereon, a strong irritant which may cause a considerable skin rash at the mere touch of the plant. Severe mezereon poisoning may constrict the larynx and lead to violent choking. Because of these torturous properties, the plant is known by various picturesque names in the herblores of some countries, such as Bottleneck, etc.

Dichroa febrifuga—Huang ch'ang shan
The infusion prepared from the root of the herb is a well-known and time-proven antiperiodic for malaria.

*Ephedra sinica—Ma huang—*Chinese Ephedra (Horsetail)
The excellent curative power of Ma huang in the treatment of pulmonary diseases has been known to the Chinese since time immemorial. It is also suggested as a diaphoretic, and is administered as an expectorant in cases of persistent coughs and bronchitis; also used for various inflammations of the nasal membrane (rhinitis, coryza), for fever and breathing difficulties, blocked-up ears, retention of urine, dropsy, headaches, and to clear up the exudations of eye inflammations.

Ephedra is one of the major sources of natural ephedrine.

For that reason, it is one of those medicinal herbs that have found unanimous acclaim during "scientific" eras. Ephedrine can no longer be omitted from the list of Western pharmacological remedies, especially not from the remedies used in the treatment of asthmatic attacks. According to reliable sources, *Ma huang* has been known and used for at least 5,000 years in China, but its fortunes in the West have fluctuated. In 1887 it was introduced to medical science by the Japanese Nagai as a mydriatic (to dilate the pupils) in the treatment of eye diseases. But soon thereafter it fell into disuse and was forgotten, until it was rediscovered in 1925, this time, though, as a medicament for asthmatic ailments. During all this, folk medicine and some off-the-track practitioners have always been loyal to the herb and its powers.

Epimedium macranthum—Yin yang ts'ao—Longspur Epimedium (species of Barrenwort)

A splendid means—to the Chinese—of enhancing a man's sexual potency; supposed to increase sperm; furthers fertility and has a general restoring and stimulating effect on the whole body (as most aphrodisiacs do).

Eucommia ulmoides—Tu chung—species of Rubber Tree

Tu chung is a good diuretic and restorative. The leaves are used in the treatment of hemorrhoids.

Euphorbia esula L.—Ta chi—Leafy Spurge (Wolf's Milk)

Induces evacuation of bowels and bladder; cures the twelve types of dropsy, acute pains, abscesses in the neck or the armpit, and swollen legs; vasodilator (dilates the blood vessels).

Euphorbia lathyris L.—Hsü sui tze—Caper Spurge

Very effective for dropsy, ulcers of various kinds, and swellings.

The leafy spurge is poisonous. People who have tried it as medicine by eating the seeds or using them in enemas have been known to meet with a fatal end. No research exists (in Europe, at any rate) on the medical efficacy of the plant, or on proper dosages. The caper spurge, on the other hand, was used as a cathartic, although no actual purgative ingredients have been detected in the plant; but it does contain some other, rather virulent substances. Other species of *Euphorbia* have yielded medicines for asthma and other respiratory affections, angina pectoris, and several other dis-

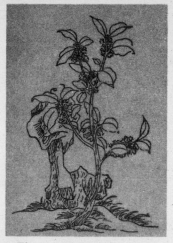

Fig. 6. *Cinnamomum cassia*
Cinnamon.

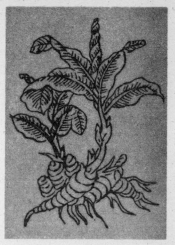

Fig. 7. *Curcuma longa*
Turmeric.

Fig. 8. *Centiana scabra*
Rough Gentian.

Fig. 9. *Nelumbium speciosum*
Lotus Flower.

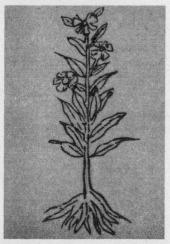

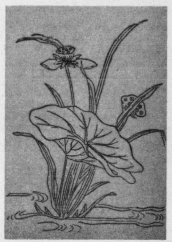

eases. In Europe, *Euphorbia lathyris* is no longer used medicinally.

*Foeniculum vulgare—Hui hsiang—*Common Fennel
Promotes digestion, cures eye catarrhs and is recommended as a "rupture medicine" for hernias.

*Forsythia suspensa—Lian ch'iao—*Weeping Forsythia
Destroys intestinal worms; relieves pain when urinating; cures swellings.

*Fritillaria imperialis—Pei mu—*Imperial Fritillary (Crown Imperial)
Pei mu is said to be highly effective for inflammation in the throat, for fever, rheumatism, coughs, and eye affections; its curative powers are enhanced by combining the herb with dried orange rinds and sugar.

The crown imperial, native to the region from Iran to the Himalayan mountain range, is considered merely an ornamental garden favorite in the West. The bulb of the plant contains a poison affecting the heart, but loses its toxin when boiled.

*Gentiana scabra—Lung tan ts'ai—*Rough Gentian
Removes cold as well as heat from the bones; strengthens the stomach; employed in cases of eye diseases, swollen and aching feet, and ulcers.

Various types of gentian have always been esteemed as restoratives, febrifuges, and as improvers of the appetite, and are so recommended in old herbals; the root is used medicinally.

*Glycine Soja—Ta tou—*Soy Bean
The soy bean is one of the chief means of nourishment in China. Tou fu, a soy-bean curd, has had a reputation as a remedy for jaundice.

*Glycyrrhiza uralensis—Kan ts'ao—*species of Licorice (from the Ural)
Kan ts'ao is a pain-reliever, dilates the blood vessels, and builds up blood; it settles the stomach and strengthens spleen and lungs; also said to have a cooling effect, especially in cases of high fever, and is an important admixture in many composite medications.

*Hydnocarpus anthelmintica—Ta feng tze—*Common (Chinese) Chaulmoogra

*The oil extracted from this herb reputedly cures leprosy
and all kinds of open wounds; also neutralizes poison.*

*Inula britannica—Hsün fu hua—*British Inula (Elecampane)
*Makes for brisk blood circulation; removes congestions
and swellings due to intestinal dropsy; cures neuralgias in
head and eyes; serves as an expectorant in the case of obstinate, deep-seated coughs; and is soothing as a salve for
pulled muscles and fractures.*

*Juglans regia—Hu t'ao—*Persian Walnut
*Walnuts exert an invigorating effect on kidneys and stom-
ach; also used to the same end in the West.*

*Kaempferia galanga—Shan nai—*Capoor Cutchery (dried
root of Indian species of Resurrection Lily)
*Makes for good blood circulation and achieves excellent
curative results with boils and purulent teeth.*

Leonurus sibiricus—I mu ts'ao or *Chung wei tze—*Siberian
Motherwort
*As its name suggests, this herb is a favorite medication
for gynecological diseases and disorders; used in the treatment of menstrual complaints, excessive bleeding, vaginal
discharge, and dropsy; is also supposed to ameliorate headaches, heavy feeling in the limbs, and congestions of all
kinds; besides enabling women to conceive, it improves
man's virility and fertility.*

Motherwort, of the mint family, was used for the same
purposes in Europe. Paracelsus listed the common motherwort as *Cordiaca,* recommending it as a sedative for heart
palpitation, an antispasmodic for diaphragm spasms, and
apparently also as a stomach-settler. A herbal of the year
1485 refers to the fact that Dioscorides Pedanius (who in
the first century A.D. described some 600 plants in his work
on medical botany) had already suggested the use of the
common motherwort (*Cordiaca*) as a remedy for gastric
affections.

It has been claimed repeatedly that the common motherwort has a tranquilizing effect similar to that of valerian
essence. However, the presence of an active substance with
that quality has not yet been ascertained in the *Leonurus
herb*—at least not to the time of this writing.

*Liriope spicata—Mai men tung—*Lilyturf
Cures nausea and dyspnea (short-windedness).

Mahonia ganpinnensis Fedde—La huang po—species of the Barberry (Berberis) Family
Mitigates severe toothache.

Malva verticellata—Tung kuei tze—Cluster Mallow
Promotes the flux of urine (diuretic), and relieves indigestion.

Morus tartarica—San ken—Russian Mulberry Tree
The inner rinds of the mulberry root are used in the treatment of swellings; said to be of beneficial effect also in cases of cancerous ulcers.

Myristica fragrans—Jou tou k'ou—Common Nutmeg
Curative effect on cardiac affections, and a carminative; serves excellently as a flavoring agent in milk for children who refuse to drink it plain.
The oil of the nutmeg contains the glyceride myristin, which may cause poisoning and miscarriages when administered in large doses.

Nauclea sinensis Oliv.—Tiao t'eng tiao—species of the Fathead Tree Family
Cures attacks of vertigo and scintillations before the eyes.

Nelumbrium speciosum—Lien tze—Lotus Flower
The leaves of the lotus are used in making fever-reducing preparations; applied externally, they heal eczema and minor skin ulcers.

Nephelium litchi—Li chih—Chinese Litchi
The fruits of the Nephelium litchi *serve as a tonic. Repeated attempts have been made to cultivate these extremely aromatic fruits in Europe and America, but have failed so far.*

Nephelium longana Camb.—Lung yen—Dragon-Eyes (*Euphoria longan*)
It is strongly recommended that the fruits of the Lung yen *be taken when one is confronted with serious mental or intellectual problems; they are regarded as stimulating to the intellect and invigorating to the entire body.*

Oryza—Mi—Rice
Steamed rice is not only the basic means of subsistence for the Chinese, but is also reputed to restore bad hearing and weakened eyes, as well as to quench thirst.

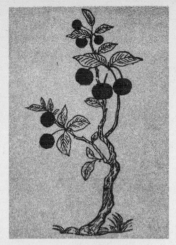

Fig. 10. *Nephelium litchi*
Litchi fruits.

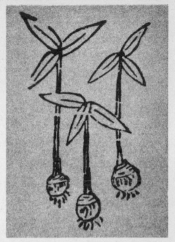

Fig. 11. *Pinellia tuberifera.*

Fig. 12. *Quisqualis sinensis.*

Fig. 13. *Rehmannia glutinosa.*

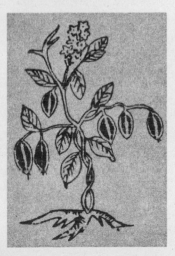

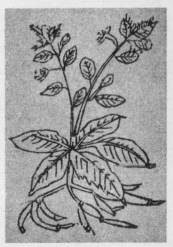

Pachyma cocos—Fu ling
Fu ling *is used in treating edema and diarrhea; it regulates urine discharge, mitigates heart pangs, restores and refreshes body and mind, and prolongs life.*

*Paeonia albiflora Pall.—P'ai shao—*Chinese (White) Peony
Supposedly effective in all afflictions connected with pregnancy and childbirth.

*Paeonia moutan—Mu tan—*Tree Peony
Since the peony is considered the queen of flowers, it is only fitting that it should be endowed with healing powers of royal dimensions; the rind is furthermore used as a subsidiary ingredient in tonic preparations.

*Peucedamum decursivum—Ch'ien hu—*species of Hogfennel
Cures coughs; dispels fever; effective against cholera.
The masterwort, a close relative of the *Peucedamum officinale* (common hogfennel), is highly esteemed in folk medicine even today as having great medicinal value, not only for coughs and hoarseness, but also for apoplectic attacks and several other afflictions. Successful results have also been claimed in cases of rheumatism and gout, and even in delirium tremens. Even if most of these properties are obviously wishful thinking, a closer exploration of the medicinal qualities of the masterwort may be profitable.

Pinellia tuberifera—Pan hsia
Helps to relieve headaches, feelings of dizziness, and emotional oppression; acts as a tonic and excitant.

*Pinus—Sung—*Pine Tree
The needles of the pine tree are used in fumigating the home to aid the expulsion of evil spirits; an aromatic tea may be prepared from the cones.

*Pistacia lentiscus L.—Ju hsiang—*Lentisk Pistachio
The pistachio produces the mastic from which plasters and poultices are prepared.

*Plantago major—Che ch'ien tze—*Rippleseed Plantain
A diuretic; said to increase sperm and fertility; soothes coughs and lends an intense glow to the eyes.
The mucilage contained in the various species of plantain is probably the reason for its use as an emollient for coughs

and sore throats. According to laboratory tests, one of the species, the ribwort (*Plantago lanceolata*), contains a substance that prevents blood-coagulation.

Platycodon grandiflorum—Chieh keng—Balloon Flower
Effective for eye inflammations, aching throats, toothache and dry coughs, as well as flatulence.

Polygala tenuifolia—Yuan chih—species of Milkwort (or Snakeroot)
Improves vision and hearing; cures lapses of memory and aids concentration.

Polygonatum falcatum—Huang ching—species of Solomon's Seal
Invigorating effect on heart, muscles, lungs, and bones; counted among the life-prolonging herbs.

Polygonum aviculare—Pien hsü—Prostrate Knotweed
Cleanses the urine; relieves abdominal pains; destroys intestinal worms; very curative results in affections of the lungs and in jaundice.

Besides tannin, mucilage, and minor amounts of volatile oils, the knotweed contains salicic acid, which would account for its persistence in folk medicine as a medication for lung diseases. Plants containing salicic acid are to this day used in the treatment of chronic pulmonary tuberculosis.

Polygonum barbatum—Mao liao—species of Knotweed
An ointment made from the leaves and stems of this knotweed is used for cancer.

Polygonum multiflorum Thunb.—Ho shou niao—Tuber Fleeceflower
Restores strength to liver, muscles, and bones; increases sperm; produces fertility; abates fever; cures obstinate ulcers.

Prunus Persica—T'ao—Peach
The stones of peaches are used in treating rheumatism and constipation.

The oil contained in the seeds of the peach, *oleum persicarum*, is medicinal and is used more or less for the same purposes as oil of bitter almond. Its active ingredient—amygdalin—is also inherent in the tree's leaves. Amygdalin is a glucoside of prussic acid, or hydrocyanic acid, which is one of the most virulent toxins known to man. When a person swallows prussic acid, he collapses with a shriek—released by the sudden spasm of the musculature—and dies instantly. Poisoning caused by bitter almonds or peach stones, which occurs repeatedly, especially with children, naturally takes a slower course. The prussic-acid components impede the work of the respiratory enzymes; the nervous system is impaired; agony and palpitations of the heart are the result. The poisoned person may be saved, if the respiration can be kept flowing.

Amygdalin was formerly prescribed, mainly in the form of oil of bitter almond, as a demulcent for sore throats and as a pain-reliever. Since then, a number of less virulent and more efficient drugs have been developed, and medicinal science has virtually discontinued the use of oil of bitter almond.

Psoralea corylifolia—P'o ku chih—Malay-Tea Scurf Pea
Said to intensify the sexual powers; removes menstrual disorders; effective against sensations of chilliness and pains in the lower back and the knees.

Punica granatum—An shih liu—Pomegranate
The bark of the pomegranate tree is employed in arresting diarrhea.
The bark contains tannin, resin, and various sugar substances; several alkaloids have also been discovered. The alkaloids explain the anthelmintic (worm-killing) properties of the bark, especially in the case of tapeworms. The tannin substances account for the use in diarrhea cases. The most potent medicinal part is the skin of the tree's roots.

Quisqualis sinensis and *Quisqualis indica—Shih chün tze—Quisqualis indica* is the Rangoon Creeper
Excellent vermifuge (expellant of intestinal worms). Administered to children after the consumption of undue amounts of candy.

Rehmannia glutinosa—Ti huang
Remedy for heart attacks, hemorrhages, and burning of the feet.

Rhamnus purshiana DC.—Mei shu li—Cascara Buckthorn
Purgative; main active ingredients are emodins, which are also present in the species *Cascara sagrada*, the American buckthorn. No essential difference in the efficacy between the American and the European buckthorn has been determined.

*Rheum officinale—Ta huang—*Rhubarb, medicinal
In China, also, the rhubarb is held in esteem as a means of alleviating constipation. It is furthermore used in the treatment of dropsy, purulent ulcers, fever, coughs, hoarseness, and diseases of the heart.

*Ricinus communis—Pi ma tze—*Castor Bean
Has a laxative effect; cures tongue swellings and ulcers; removes speech disturbances and hearing difficulties.

*Salix purpurea L.—Ch'uan liu—*Purple Willow
The bark of the tree serves as an admixture in a prescription for rheumatism.

*Salvia miltiorrhiza L.—Tan shen—*species of Sage
Allays fever; renews the blood; cures gynecological diseases, as well as eye diseases.

*Saponaria vaccaria—Wang pu liu hsing—*Cow Soapwort
Vasodilator; stimulates the blood circulation; heals wounds caused by weapons; serves to remove thorns, wood, or bamboo splinters from the flesh; but is dangerous for pregnant women.

*Schisandra sinensis—Wu wei tze—*Chinese Magnolia
Very effective remedy for urinary and renal complaints.

*Scrophularia oldhami Yüan shen—*species of Figwort
Soothes coughing and aching throats, cures scrofula and fever; encourages bowel movement and urination; strengthens the eyes.

Stemona sessifolia—Po p'u
Used for fever and coughs, as well as to prevent the forming of pus.

*Taraxacum officinale L.—P'u kung yin—*Common Dandelion (Leontodon)
Cures mammillary ulcers; disperses fever; used in treating venereal diseases; neutralizes toxins within the body.

*Thea sinensis—Ch'a—*Common (Chinese) Tea
Many Chinese physicians maintain that tea has specific therapeutic properties. The black bohea tea from the province of Fukien, besides being an exceptionally aromatic beverage, is thought to possess particularly effective healing powers. In most tea-growing regions, great care is taken that

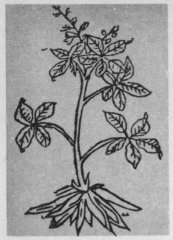

Fig. 14. *Salvia miltiorrhiza L.*
Sage.

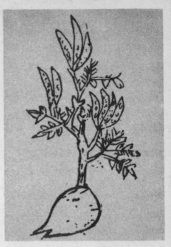

Fig. 15. *Trigonella fœnum-
græcum*
Trigonella (Fenugreek).

Fig. 16. *Tremella fuciformis*
Tremella fungus.

Fig. 17. *Zingiber officinale*
Common Ginger.

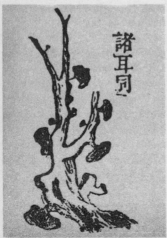

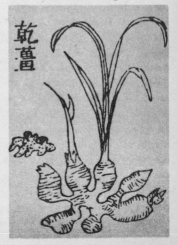

the tea leaves are gathered early in the morning, when they are still moist and glistening with the morning dew. Leaves that are picked just after the first thunderstorm of the year are said to be of especially good medicinal quality. Such tea is recommended for treating colds, headaches, flatulence, dysentery, coughing, and weakness of the eyes (which might be explained by the stimulated blood circulation). To alleviate constipation, it is suggested that one drink an infusion made of tea leaves twisted into pills and then boiled in onion water. Tea is often flavored with Chu lan, Chloranthus inconspicua.

The origin of the tea plant is ascribed to an ancient myth which in its own way throws a merciless spotlight on the brutality of Old Chinese punishments. A delinquent was sentenced to have his eyelids cut off—a measure that is bound to lead to blindness because of the drying out of the conjunctiva and the cornea. However, the legend goes that the poor wretch was innocent of the crime, and when the executioner performed his cruel task and the defendant's severed eyelids dropped to the ground, the bud of a plant—a tea plant—shot out of that very spot in the earth and began to grow. If nothing else, the story reveals that the ancient Chinese were well aware of the sleep-denying properties of the tea plant, caused by one of its constituents, the alkaloid caffeine (theine). Tannin, another of the leaves' substances, was formerly used to stop diarrhea.

Tremella fuciformis—Mu erh
A fungus growing on decayed elms and oak trees; said to have therapeutic properties for pulmonary diseases.

Trigonella fœnum-græcum—Hu lu pa—Fenugreek (Trigonella)
Very commonly used to loosen phlegm in air ducts, and as a restorative.

Veratrum nigrum—Li lu—Black False Hellebore
Effective emetic for swallowed poisons; also causes sneezing.

Verbena officinalis—Ma pien ts'ao—European Verbena
Popular antiperiodic for malaria, and vermifuge.

Zingiber officinale—Chiang—Common Ginger
Settles nauseous stomach and dyspepsia; strengthens the heart.

Zizyphus vulgaris—Tsao—Common Jujube (Chinese Date)

Supports heart and lung functions and tones up blood circulation; dries up excessive mucus and restores strength to a generally enfeebled body.

The Story of the Poppy

*Papaver somniferum—P'ai hua ying su—*Opium Poppy

Opium! Song of the inscrutable Orient, of adventure and of depravity, dim red light and the stench of smoke in murky Chinese taverns, and the hero dashing in tearing his drugged friend—or perchance a fair lady—from the clutches of evil!

Yes, to the Western mind the vice of opium smoking is inextricably connected with China. Yet opium is a comparative latecomer in China's history. It is first mentioned in medical books around A.D. 1000, and even then merely as a specific for diarrhea. It was only in the mid-seventeenth century, when Ch'ung Ch'en, the last emperor of the Ming Dynasty, chanced upon the unfortunate idea of prohibiting the smoking of tobacco, that opium, introduced from the Near East and Africa, became a far more dangerous compensation.

Long before that, Egyptians and Europeans had made bad use of the poppy seed by giving it to children as a pacifier; it is thought that Paracelsus, who lived around 1500, was addicted to opium; and the health of some peoples in the Near East had already been severely damaged by the intoxicant, while the opium dens in Mecca were still plying a flourishing business.

It is true, however, that once in China, the vice spread with inordinate force and rapidity. This may have been due partly to a racial phenomenon, for different races show different reactions to the alkaloids contained in opium. A white person—even a morphine addict—when under the toxin's influence, is lifted into a rosy, beatific world where all his anxieties are dissipated; but this is where it ends, as a rule. When a member of an oriental race inhales opium, he has distinctly erotic hallucinations. The "houris of the Seven Heavens" flutter around him alluringly, and he is capable of experiencing such voluptuous joys as his waking self could never imagine.

Whether morphine addict of the West or opium smoker of the East, all drug takers know only too well that the poison will gradually destroy their bodies and that they will pay for their dreams of rapture with creeping misery and a pitiful end. But such knowledge is futile, because it is the very essence of the addiction that the powers of resistance decline progressively, despite the intellect's better reasoning.

There were a number of sensible minds in China who undertook to curb the evil by trying to prevent the import of opium. But European mercantile ambitions, and undoubtedly Chinese too to some extent, proved stronger. When Emperor Tao Kuang in 1840 moved to extinguish the opium pipes once for all, he only managed to hasten the final disaster: the outbreak of war between England and China. The Opium War was to deprive China of much of its territory, and the statutes of the subsequent treaty gave virtually free license to the unrestricted import of the poisonous drug.

Today the growing and marketing of the opium poppy is internationally controlled. For medical purposes alone, 330,-000 kilograms (approximately 733,300 pounds) are needed annually; but how much more is secretly harvested in the hidden areas of Asia and other parts of the world is anybody's guess.

The opium prepared for smoking, *Chandu* or *Yen Kao* in Chinese, is a darkish, pliable mass that burns away in the pipe with a lingering glow. The drug is obtained by cutting slits in the unripe seed capsule of the poppy; a milky-white sap oozes out, which is gathered and left to dry. Since the poppy capsules found in ancient lake dwellings of Europe bear traces of such incisions, it is generally concluded that opium was known during the lake-dweller period (see table of dates, below).

Twenty-five per cent of the content of opium consists of alkaloids, the most significant of which is morphine. Its secondary alkaloid is codeine, widely known as a medicine for chronic coughs and as a subsidiary ingredient in other medications. Ripe poppy seeds are non-poisonous, and equally harmless are the wild poppies frequently found growing as weeds in fields and meadows.

IMPORTANT DATES IN THE HISTORY OF OPIUM

Ancient Egypt, from Papyrus	Poppy juice employed as sleeping drug for children.
2000 B.C.	From this period date the capsules with the typical incisions found in the Swiss lake dwellings (Lake Constance).

800 B.C.	Homer, in Book IV of the *Odyssey:* Helen of Troy, (now back in Argos) entertaining the son of Odysseus, Telemachus, slips into his cup of wine a drug that has the power of robbing grief and anger of their sting and banishing painful memories. She had received this anodyne (presumably opium) from an Egyptian lady.
A.D. 47	Scribonius Largus, Roman pharmacologist, describes the value of opium as a medication in *Compositiones Medicamentorum,* a collection of 271 prescriptions. (This is the earliest account of the preparation of opium for medical purposes.)
Early 1500's	Theophrastus Bombastus Paracelsus von Hohenheim (Swiss alchemist and physician, 1493?–1541) "brings back" into medical therapy an opium derivative that he praises highly—*laudanum.* Historians claim that Paracelsus himself was addicted to opium.
1628–1644	Ch'ung Ch'en, the last emperor of the Ming Dynasty, forbids the smoking of tobacco. Opium begins to take its place.
1699	The British physician Thomas Sydenham (1624–1689), known as the English Hippocrates, praises opium and introduces it to the British Isles.
1806	The German apothecary Sertürner (born 1783 at Paderborn) isolates the principal and most crucial alkaloid, morphine, from opium.
1840–1842	Emperor Tao Kuang prohibits the import of opium and orders all foreign merchants to demolish their storehouses. The result is the Opium War, which in turn results in the inglorious Peace of Shanghai. Among other conditions forced upon China are the surrender of Hong Kong to England and laws granting special rights to alien merchants ("the foreign devils").
1917	A powerful anti-opium campaign leads to the destruction of large stocks of opium in China.

Human, Animal, and Mineral "Medicines"

Along with herbs and plants, the Chinese esteemed a number of other pharmaceuticals, some of which were also known in ancient and medieval Europe. Most of them are —to put it mildly—unappetizing concoctions. But before we deride them as disgusting nonsense, let us not forget that during the recent World Wars I and II, urine was used in cases of emergency. Soldiers would apply the urine to their wounds as a disinfectant and healing agent—the urine of a healthy person is completely free of germs! The treatment of slow-healing wounds with urea (the soluble nitrogenous substance of urine) often produces excellent results and is employed within the field of scientific medicine. A related example may be the use of boys' urine in the treatment of pulmonary tuberculosis, a domestic remedy that is kept alive stubbornly in the folk-medicines even of Western countries. It must be mentioned here that no conclusive results of experiments with urea or any other urine extractive have been available to the authors.

With the above as a background, it will not be too shocking to learn that the Chinese used all possible bodily secretions for their medicaments. Again, may we point out that in Europe also menstrual blood (hormone content!) was once used as a regular ingredient of love potions.

The following is a small section of such exotic "cures"; may it suffice as a sample offering.

Elephant Skin *(Hsiang p'i):* The ashes of burnt elephant skin close slow-healing wounds.

Shark Fins *(Sha ch'i)* are a delectable seafood and are said to restore strength. Their preparation takes several days. On the first day they are cooked slightly longer than an hour and are then left to cool in the liquid; on the next day they are boiled again for a while and left to cool; and so on, until the flesh is a pure white and the gray skin can be peeled off easily.

Deer Antlers *(Lu kung)* strengthen the bones. An excellent excitant for men whose sexual potency is declining. They also dispel nightmares and the ghosts participating in them.

Honey *(Mi tang)* is used profusely in Chinese medicine, especially as a binding agent in the preparation of pills.

Lime—Calcium *(Shih hui)* is used for excessive mucus.

Boys' Urine *(T'ung pien)* is said to possess great curative power in the case of lung diseases. Swallowed warm, it is said to remove hoarseness and soothe inflamed throats. Also very popular as a tonic and as a solvent for clogged blood vessels in pregnant women. It is to be taken three times a day, warm, mixed with a dash of wine.

Toads *(Ch'an):* The skin secretion of toads used externally is said to be a fine cure for dog bites. The blood of toads mixed with sugar will extract swallowed iron objects from the stomach when imbibed immediately after the accident.

Dragonflies *(Chin t'ing)* are counted among the love-medicines, since they reputedly intensify sexual vigor. Several sources recommend them as a cooling agent for inflammations. If the heads of dragonflies are buried in the house on the fifth day of the fifth month, their eyes will be transformed into blue pearls.

Quicksilver—Mercury *(Shui yin)* is employed externally to treat venereal diseases.

Rhinoceros Horn *(Hsi chio)* is highly effective when applied to pus boils (furuncles). It is also prescribed as an antitoxin for snake bites.

Turtle Shells *(Kuei pei)* are used as an emulgent to stimulate weak kidneys; will also remove gallstones.

Snake Flesh *(She jou),* also highly appreciated as a delicacy, keeps eyes healthy and vision clear.

Snuff *(Pi yen):* Snuff was first introduced into China around 1660 and quickly became as much a fashion there as it was in Europe. While snuff takers in the West were fond of their little boxes of gold and silver, or rare wood, the Chinese preferred dainty flasks. Within a short time an entirely new craft had developed, devoted solely to the creation of artfully shaped and decorated snuff *flacons.* The tobacco was lifted out with tiny wooden spoons, and the lid was either a beautiful piece of coral or a stopper carved from semiprecious gems. In spite of this, the snuffing fad was short-lived in China; soon it succumbed to the rising popularity of waterpipe-smoking.

Swallows' Nests *(Yen wo),* another coveted delicacy, are used as a reviving remedy for old or sickly people. Since swallows build their nests with certain algae and grasses that are exceedingly rich in vitamins, the belief in their medicinal value is probably not too far-fetched.

Pig's Blood *(Chu hsüeh)* is an extremely strengthening liquid after spells of weakness and severe illnesses, but should be shunned by pregnant women.

Pig's Kidneys *(Chu shen)* ease pains in the back and temper ear inflammations.

Lard *(Chu chi)*, mixed with roasted onions and rubbed on the chest, is excellent for loosening deep-seated coughs. Beyond that, it speeds the healing of wounds and ejects poison from the stomach.

Seahorses *(Hai ma)*, pulverized, are said to cure goiters.

Cuttlefish—Sepia *(Wu tse):* Its ink, mixed with vinegar, is said to ameliorate heart conditions.

A most awesome medication—to the non-Chinese—is the one that requires the cooking of a soup from one's own flesh. Since ancient times in Chinese history, it has never been a rare occurrence that daughters cut a piece of flesh out of their own bodies and prepared a strengthening soup from it for their sick parents, or even in-laws. If a husband is severely ill, a loving spouse may also resort to this cure. Even today such sacrifice is not unheard-of.

Chinese Love Philters

Rumor has it that sometimes in China a young man is presented with a wife—selected for him by his parents—who later turns out to be frigid. The young fellow who has met with such ill luck will find plenty of good advice in almanacs and other pertinent literature. Unfortunately, though, most of the recipes are rather difficult to carry out. Thus, the poor wretch may read that he has to obtain the brain of a monkey, wash it absolutely clear of blood and cook it with water to a thin pap. To this emulsion he must add the chopped root of the climbing herb glycine and the pulverized tips of the trembling bamboo that have already been cooked separately. This decoction is to be slipped secretly into his wife's tea; it is said to perform veritable wonders.

Of course, the impatient bridegroom has another choice. He can grind to powder the chrysanthemum stone (named after the chrysanthemum-like pattern of its veins), cook that with water to a pasty pulp and, while cooking, stir in the pulverized wings of butterflies. Then he should leave it to dry. The residue—a delicately thin layer by then—must be carefully pushed into the sleeve of the beloved without her noticing it. This charm is reported to be so potent that any resistance of the young bride will instantly be turned into joyful submission.

If the young couple want to avoid the natural offspring of the ensuing night of passionate love-making, good advice again is not far. They merely have to catch a scorpion, tear out all its feet, and roast its body to ashes. Thereupon, they must smear glue on the wings of an autumn cicada, sprinkle the scorpion ashes on it, and knead the whole matter well together. The contraceptive thus prepared is simply spread on the woman's abdomen, three fingers below the navel. Should the couple later decide that they want children, nothing will prevent it: the wife will merely have to swallow the saliva of a toad, and her fertility will be restored presently.

And what if the wife be a shrew? In that case the husband has to gather a few cobwebs, snip the mottled scars off a begonia root, and mix both together until well blended. After ten days a sediment will have formed. This has to be twisted into a small pill, which should be dropped clandestinely into her tea or meals. Now the lass will become docile and melt away with lusty desire, be she virgin or not. Caution must be preserved, however, for the drug is very virulent and should not be consumed too often, lest the conquered lady be maimed for life. The pill is said to be lethal when used five times.

To keep the external genitals young and vigorous, it is recommended that they be massaged for as long a time as the woman can hold her breath.

Another recipe reads: Take the tongues of sparrows and dry them. After seven days dip them in the saliva of a snake, simultaneously adding a spoonful of honey, which will neutralize the snake's poison. This preparation has to be swallowed at the time of intercourse; it will make the lovers seem mysteriously fascinating to one another, and it promises prolonged sexual pleasure.

If a couple wishes for especially intelligent children, these procedures have to be followed: The spouses grind to powder an oyster, mix it with the dew of flowers, and stir in ten pearls of clear and unblemished luster. As soon as day breaks, the mixture has to be put into the sunshine; at night it must stand in the moonlight. After a hundred days, dew and oyster powder will have been absorbed by the pearls. During their love-making, husband and wife each has to hold five pearls in the mouth. Children springing from such a union will burst with intelligence.

Additional valuable advice for men: Pound the shell of a male venus's-comb (a species of mollusk) to a very fine powder, add some urine, and let stand for three days, after which time put it out at noon to dry in the sun. Then dip this in donkey-water and allow it to steep another three days. Again let it dry in the noonday sun and then sprinkle it lightly with the dew of flower blossoms; this will disperse the odor of the urine. Drink from the solution at the time of copulation and you will be endowed with extraordinary potency. The potion has no undesirable aftereffects.

Or this alternative: Before falling asleep at night, put both hands between your legs, keeping them cupped around the scrotum so that the testes will never get cold. He who so proceeds from his earliest childhood onward through the rest of his life will be able to have coitus with ten women daily; and while his semen will never be exhausted, his intellect likewise will not deteriorate. He will retain a youthful virility and his hair will not become brittle.

IV

CHINESE ANATOMY

AND PHYSIOLOGY

The Body—A Sacred Gift

The great scholar Yüo Chung Tsi Ch'un had injured his foot by tripping on a stairway. For a long time after his recovery he could be seen walking about with a troubled look on his brow. His students grew anxious and worried and finally dared to inquire what the cause of their teacher's trouble might be.

Yüo Chung Tsi Ch'un replied: "Confucius, who made us aware of the sacredness of the human body, has taught us that only those shall be truly revered who at the end of their lives will return their physical bodies whole and sound. I am deeply grieved that I have not taken good care of mine, for our bodies are not our property, but a gift bequeathed to us by our parents and forebears."

The Chinese concept of the structure of the human body dominated vast areas of Asia, including the islands of Japan, and provided the foundation on which the treatment of all illnesses was based. This concept remained irrefutable dogma until the end of the nineteenth century and is even today the starting point of all medical thinking in wide regions of the East. The human organism was treated with the greatest reverence, which is the more bewildering since the life inherent in that body was apparently regarded of little value. As many tortures and other cruel punishments can be found in China's history as elsewhere in the world.

Considering the mental attitude conveyed in the above anecdote about the sacredness of the human body, it is only logical that the Chinese should have rejected surgical cuts into the living body and prohibited the dissection of corpses. As a result of such doctrines, anatomical and physiological concepts were based on speculation, or perhaps on vague notions and memories handed down from an obscure past. But need we marvel at that, when even in sixteenth-century Europe, Andreas Vesalius was prosecuted because he opened dead bodies for his anatomical studies?

The Organs

Chinese anatomy knows five "solid" organs that collect and store—the *Ts'ang*—and five "hollow" organs that excrete—the *Fu*. Beyond these, all medical books mention another organ which, for want of a better technical term, is usually translated as "warmer" in Western languages. It is said to feed the necessary life-warmth to the kidneys. Occasionally several warmers are mentioned, which are somehow connected with one another. The first warmer is located in the front part of the body, with its opening in the chest; the second one starts at the center of the chest and reaches down toward the abdomen; the third is situated within the abdominal area itself. What exactly the Old Chinese meant by the "warmer" or "warmers" is still a point of controversy.

Some scholars agree with Professor Franz Hübotter, physician and well-known sinologist, who interprets the warmers as the lymphatic system. This theory deserves at least serious consideration, since the main trunk of the lymphatic vessels—the thoracic duct—extends up through the thorax and opens into the left subclavian vein (the vein under the left clavicle), which would correspond to the opening of the first warmer in the chest.

Heart and liver were held to be the noblest and most essential organs. "My heart and my liver," whispers the Chinese lover as an especially tender endearment.

How the Chinese believed the organs to be distributed throughout the body is illustrated in figures 18 and 19, general front and back view respectively. It is quite fascinating to study these two diagrams in conjunction with the drawings following that focus on the individual organs, and to compare all of them with the European representations, figures 20 and 21, taken from the *Icones Anatomicae* of 1801–1813. The accuracy of the old Chinese concepts is remarkable.

Figures 18 and 19 picture the five *Ts'ang*-viscera—lungs, liver, spleen, heart, kidneys—and the five *Fu*-bowels—large intestine, gall bladder, stomach, small intestine, urinary bladder; figure 19 includes trachea and esophagus. True, the

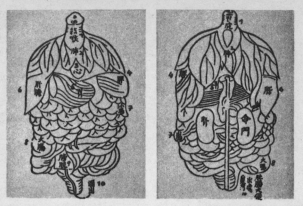

Fig. 18. (*Above left*) Chinese representation of the distribution of the organs within the human body—frontal view. Easily recognizable are: larynx (1), lungs (2), heart (3), spleen (4), stomach (5), liver (6), small intestine (7), large intestine (8), urinary bladder (9), and opening of urethra (10).

Fig. 19. (*Above right*) Representation of the distribution of the organs—dorsal view. The number (10) in this diagram indicates the anus.

Figs. 20 and 21. Representation of the distribution of the organs, frontal and dorsal views, from the anatomical plates *Icones Anatomicae,* prepared by Leopoldo Marco Antonio Caldani and his nephew Florianus Caldani, 1801–1813.

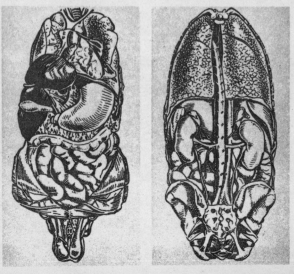

lungs are still portrayed here with six lobes, but the representation of the trachea and its branches—if this is what those forked lines indicate—is already rather close to reality. To conceive of the lungs as a six-lobed instead of five-lobed organ is surely a forgivable blunder, especially when it is counterbalanced by the relatively precise placement of the heart.

The diaphragm is very appropriately perceived as the dividing layer between the upper and lower organs. It can be seen more distinctly on figure 36.

This same diagram, 36, and the chart on page 134 and 135 testify further to the comparatively high level of anatomical knowledge. In the light of such knowledge, it will seem rather surprising that the ureters, the two thin ducts connecting the kidneys with the bladder, were completely overlooked by many Chinese anatomists.

Before going into a detailed description of the individual organs, the following general observations should be considered.

The head is the storage chamber for the essence of all knowledge. The person who walks about with his head inclined does not see the true life around him; his mind and essence will grow feeble.

The back is the storage space that houses the thorax (chest). If the back is kept bent, the condition of the shoulders will also suffer.

The loins are the storage chambers for the kidneys. If the loins are not kept springy and resilient, they will be unable to transmit movement, and the kidneys will become exhausted.

The knees are the storage chambers for the muscles. If the knees are not supple and do not bend and stretch sufficiently, a hump-back will grow and the muscles will begin to sag.

The bones are the storage chambers for the marrow. If the bones are not exercised, the joints will begin to wobble and that will wear out the bones.

The functions of the organs are compared to the various functions of government officials.

The heart is the ruler over all civil servants. From it wisdom and insight emanate.

The lungs are the administrators responsible for orderly and lawful conduct.

The liver is a general who initiates strategic operations.

The gall bladder is the leading decision-maker in the central staff.

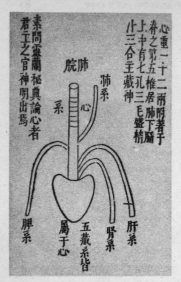

Fig. 22. Heart.

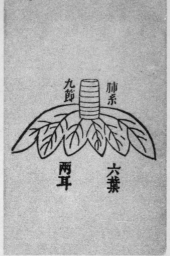

Fig. 24. Lungs.

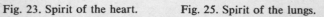

Fig. 23. Spirit of the heart.

Fig. 25. Spirit of the lungs.

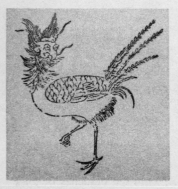

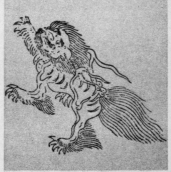

The pericardium (the sac enclosing the heart) is the ambassador bearing happiness and joy.

The spleen and stomach are sentries guarding the governmental storage rooms.

The large intestine is assigned the task of instigating evolution and changes.

The small intestine is entrusted with the execution of the changes.

The kidneys are the secretaries of labor, excelling in efficiency.

The three warmers are the officials in charge of the waterways.

The bladder is the governor of a province, who gathers the fluid secretions so that they may be channeled into their orderly positions within the pneuma, *Ch'i,* the universal spirit.

The Heart—*Hsin* (figure 22): The heart has the shape of a lotus flower, weighs 12 *liang,* and is imbedded in the center of the lungs above liver, spleen, and diaphragm. From it seven "tubes" emanate. In our diagram, one tube leads to the liver, one to a kidney, one to the spleen, and one to the lungs. In compliance with the belief in the correlation of all things, the heart is naturally connected with one of the cardinal points, the South, whose symbol is the scarlet bird. The heart therefore also resembles that bird. The spirit of the heart is *Tan Yuan,* "the core of the primordial beginning." The heart is the seat of all powers of mind and soul.

Thought of as a red organ, the heart also corresponds to fire and is, oddly enough, aligned with the small intestine. This, however, may very well be an error made by the copyists. When studying old Chinese texts and illustrations, one must always allow for such a possibility.

The Lungs—*Fei* (figure 24): The lungs weigh 3 *chin* and 3 *liang.* At the top, the breathing-gate (larynx) is located. The lungs' spirit is *Hao Hua,* "the glistening and splendid one," with the no less impressive epithet of "executor and accomplisher," and the spirit's shape is that of a tiger.

The lungs are the seat of the soul *Po,* which would largely correspond to the modern concept of the center of the nervous system (located in the brain, near the pituitary gland). The lungs are situated above the heart in the thorax and consist of six leaves (really only five "lobes," as they are called today), which end jointly in the breathing-gate.

It seems safe to assume that the anatomy of the lungs was well known to the Old Chinese, since the branches of lines

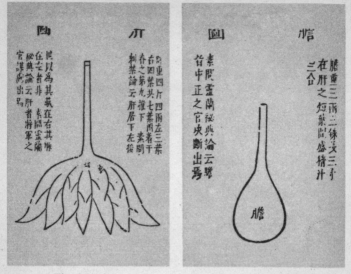

Fig. 26. Liver.

Fig. 28. Gall Bladder.

Fig. 27. Spirit of the liver.

Fig. 29. Spirit of the gall bladder.

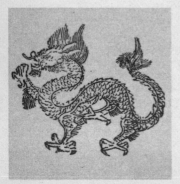

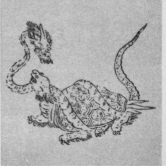

obviously indicate the network of the bronchial tubes. Nor can it be pure coincidence that the larynx is drawn in ring-like lines—they obviously represent the cricoid cartilage.

The Liver—*Kan* (figure 26): The liver weighs 4 *chin* and 4 *liang;* it consists of four leaves on the right and three leaves on the left. The shape of the liver resembles that of a hanging pumpkin. It is situated beneath the heart and is the seat of the soul *Hun*, which corresponds to the soul-concept that Western man likes to identify with the heart.

The spirit of the liver is *Lung Yen*, "dragon fumes"; its attribute, "the one who carries brightness in his mouth."

What is striking once again is the fact that the liver also is represented in the form of "leaves"—and it does, indeed, consist of lobes, as do the lungs.

The Gall Bladder—*Tan* (figure 28): The gall bladder weighs 3 *liang* and 3 *chu*, is 3 *ts'un* long and lies within the shorter leaf of the liver (it is actually lodged in a groove between the square-shaped lobe and the right lobe of the liver). It can hold 3 *ho* of liquid essence (bile). The gall bladder's spirit is *Lung Yao*, "splendor of the dragon," its epithet is "the stately and the radiant one," and its shape is that of a hybrid of turtle and snake.

The form of the gall bladder itself is aptly described as that of a hanging pumpkin. Some sources place the gall bladder more correctly "in the center of the liver."

The Stomach—*Wei* (figure 30): The stomach weighs 2 *chin* and 1 *liang*, its size is 1 *ch'ih* and 5 *ts'un*, and its diameter 5 *ts'un*.

The Old Chinese picture of the stomach is quite in tune with modern knowledge. The stomach's great expansibility is expressed in these words: "it can stretch itself until it will hold 5 *tou* of rice or 1 *tou* and 5 *sheng* of water."

The Small Intestine—*Hsiao Yang:* The circumference of the small intestine is 2½ *ts'un*, its length is 3 *chang* and 2 *ch'ih*, and its diameter 8½ *fen*.

The small intestine stretches from the spine to the navel (it fills the abdominal cavity!) and has sixteen convolutions (actually, it has an undefined number, but certainly more than sixteen).

The Large Intestine—*Ta Yang* (figure 31): Its circumference is 4 *ts'un*, and its length is 2 *chang* and 1 *ch'ih*, and its diameter is 1½ *ts'un*. It weighs 2 *chin* and 12 *liang*.

The large intestine can hold 1 *tou* of rice and 7½ *sheng* of water. It is well to point out here that whenever halves are

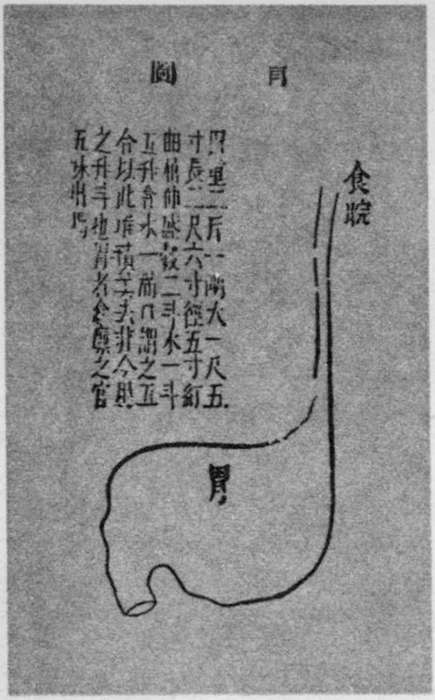

胃圖

食脘

胃

胃重二斤二兩大一尺五
寸長二尺六寸徑五寸紆
曲屈伸�受水穀三斗五
升其中之穀二斗水一斗
五升而滿上焦泄氣出其
精微慓悍滑疾下焦下溉
諸腸

Fig. 30. Stomach.

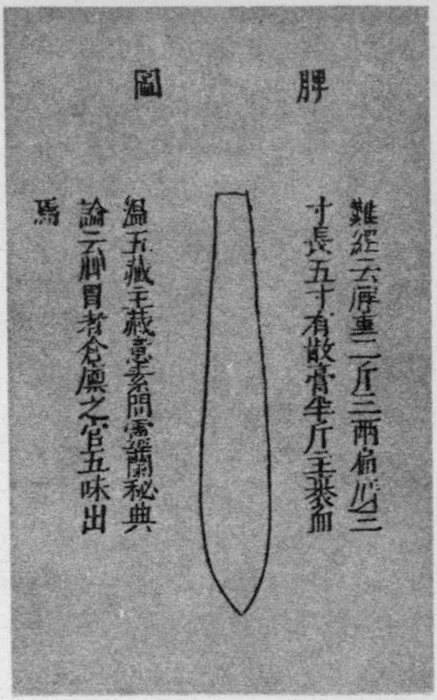

脾圖

馬

難經云厚重二斤三兩偏廣三
寸長五寸有散膏半斤主裹血

溫五臟主藏意素問靈蘭秘典
論云脾胃者倉廩之官五味出
焉

Fig. 32. Spleen.

Fig. 31. Large Intestine.

Fig. 33. Spirit of the spleen.

大腸圖

大腸接小腸為直腸
陰遺肛膀直腸
即肛門乃

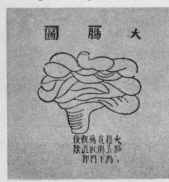

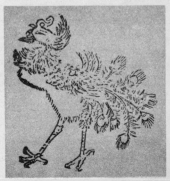

mentioned, such as one-half *sheng*, the Chinese spoke of a smaller half and a larger half.*

The Spleen—*P'i* (figure 32): The spleen weighs 2 *chin* and 3 *liang*, is 3 *ts'un* wide and 5 *ts'un* long.

This organ has always been rather mysterious. Every medical student knows the story of the State medical examination, which is told of many famous professors. Trembling nervously, the candidate stutters: "I am . . . I am terribly sorry, Professor, I can assure you that I knew the function of the spleen only this morning. . . . I am just so excited that it has completely slipped my mind." "For Heaven's sake, young man," bellows out the professor, "think hard! Try with all your might to remember it; for you are the only person in the world who knew it!"

Until fairly recently, practically nothing was known of the function of the spleen, and even today our knowledge is still limited. The Old Chinese must have been just as helpless. If most other organs were visualized and transmitted to paper with fair exactitude, the spleen remains a veritable painting of fantasy. Nonetheless, it is fairly accurately placed above the navel and behind the stomach, and its shape is not badly characterized as "a cup turned upside down."

The spleen's spirit is identified with the phoenix. It bears the name *Ch'ang Tsai*, "the one who dwells here forever," which adds nothing, of course, that enlightens us on the spleen's function. One is tempted to suspect the Chinese of the same subterfuge that Western science has often been accused of: "If thou knowest not enough about a thing, give it a name that will ring well in the ear."

The Kidneys—*Shen* (figure 34): One kidney weighs 1 *chin* and 2 *liang*. Both lie opposite the navel, at the level of the fourteenth spinal disk. (The actual position of the kidneys is variable; the left one usually lies somewhat higher than the right one. Yet, they do, indeed, both lie in the vicinity of the fourteenth "disk.") Each kidney measures 1½ *ts'un*. Many Chinese authors imagine that urine is passed from the small intestine into the bladder "at the point where that intestine touches the bladder."

---

* Western students of Old Chinese works and indexes are continually irritated by the lack of system in the recording of numbers. Granted that to the Old Chinese it was all very clear and systematic, one thing becomes evident upon talking to Chinese physicians and scientists: modern Chinese are just as confounded by their forefathers' numerical trickeries.

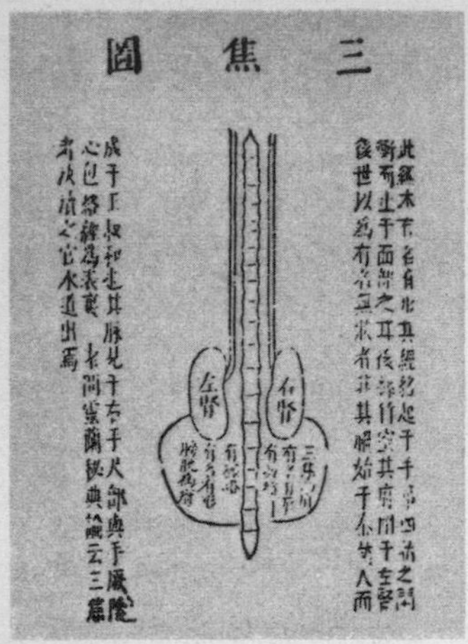

三焦圖

左腎　右腎

Fig. 34. Kidneys and "Warmers."

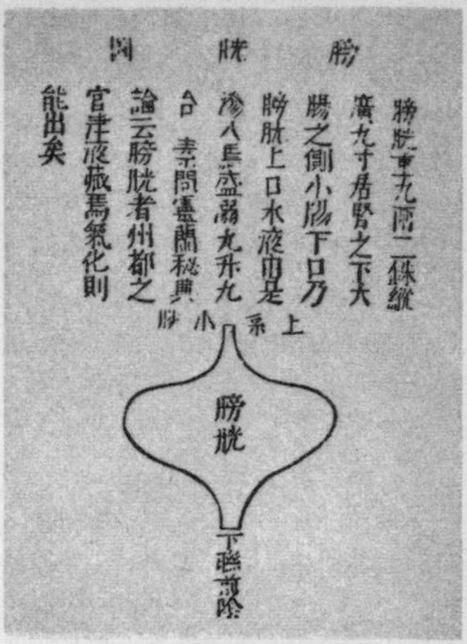

膀胱圖

膀胱

下極之闊

Fig. 35. Urinary Bladder.

Fig. 36. Location of viscera and intestines, side view:

1) *Ko,* diaphragm
2) *Kan,* liver
3) Lobe of liver close to *Tai Yang*
4) Lobe of liver close to *Tai Yin*
5) *Wei,* stomach
6) *P'i,* spleen
7) *Ming Men* (Door of Life), kidney
8) *Hsiao Yang,* small intestine
9) *Ta Yang,* large intestine
10) *Kang men,* anus
11) *Pang Kuang,* bladder
12) *Ni Ch'u,* "water opening" (urethra)

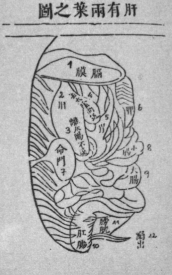

肝有兩葉之圖

膈膜
命門子
膀胱
肛腸
漏出

Although the location of the kidneys was an incontestable fact for Chinese physicians, their function could not be agreed upon. While some texts subscribe to the theory that the urine is created in the kidneys, others are unaware of any connection between the kidneys and the urinary process. When not completely ignored, the ureters are interpreted either as ligaments winding around the intestines, or as tubes transporting the male semen.

That the kidneys were closely connected with procreation is apparent from figure 19, where the right kidney—of the male body—is designated "door of life." It was believed that the semen was stored in it, and only the left kidney was considered an "intestinal" kidney—it alone was credited with producing urine, at least by some scholars. The right kidney in the female body was believed to be connected with motherhood.

The spirit of the kidneys is *Hsüan Yen*, "black darkness." It is symbolized by a two-headed stag.

The Three Warmers—*San Chiao* (figure 34): As pointed out before, the exact significance of these "organs" has not been established, although various explanations have been put forward, notably the one by Professor Hübotter, who interprets the warmers as the lymphatic system.* Whatever its meaning, the warmer is indicated in figure 34 by the circular line connecting the right kidney (*yu shen*) with the left kidney (*tso shen*).

The Bladder—*Pang Kuang* (figure 35): The bladder weighs 9 *liang* and 2 *chu* and has a diameter of 9 *ts'un*. It can hold 9 *sheng* and 9 *ho* of water and is situated below the kidneys and next to the lower orifice of the small intestine (at the point where the small intestine becomes the large intestine, i.e., where the appendix protrudes from the beginning of the large intestine). The urine enters through an opening at the top of the bladder—from the small intestine, it should be remembered! That many theorists held to this opinion is clear from figure 36: the "organ" numbered 12, which at first glance appears to be the appendix, reveals itself as the "water opening" upon closer study. Or is this one of those copyist's blunders? It is hard to determine this now, when the Old Chinese had such conflicting ideas about the urinary tracts.

* *Chinesisch-Tibetische Pharmakologie*, Ulm, 1957.

The Seasons and Their Relationship to the

Inner Organs

As we have learned, the sacred human body was believed to be a link in the harmonious workings of the cosmos, and as such was subject to all the laws of nature, to her periods of ripening and decaying, to the heat of the sun and the cold of the winds. As a logical consequence, each organ within the body corresponded to a certain season.

The heart is the ruler over the summer. Heart pulse and the pulse of the small intestine are closely connected. If the heart needs treatment, the acupuncture points of the small intestine will therefore have to be treated simultaneously. The heart is the root of life and generates all changes in the spirit. The condition of the heart may be read from a person's complexion. The heart fills the blood vessels and feeds life to the pulses.

The lungs are rulers over the autumn. Since the lungs correspond to the large intestine, both organs have to be treated together. The lungs are the stronghold and the root of the breath. Their condition manifests itself in the skin and body-hair (the pale skin of tubercular people may have been responsible for this theory).

The liver is ruler over the spring. It is the root of life's ultimate action; its condition is revealed in the finger and toe nails as well as in the muscles.

Small intestine, large intestine, spleen, and warmer are the storage chambers within the body (and are therefore often referred to as receptacles). Their condition may be read from a person's lips; if injured, they cause whiteness in the region of the mouth. They act upon flesh and muscles and belong to that essence of *Yin* which penetrates through the aura of the earth.

The spleen is ruler over the end of summer, which is conceived of as a season by itself (see table of Correspondencies in Chapter I).

The kidneys are rulers over the winter. Kidneys and bladder are related and have to be treated as one in acupuncture. Within the kidneys, "essence" is stored, and they govern all that is secluded and dormant and that is hoarded up. Their condition is disclosed in bones and head-hair.

Throat, larynx, chest, and ribs are only indirectly connected with the seasons and are therefore little susceptible to the influences of the winds.

At first glance, this pronouncement may seem surprisingly contradictory to common experience—icy winds being likely contributors to sore throats, etc. But catarrhs are probably not meant here. Instead, the "winds" referred to may be the hot, sultry winds, such as the foehn of the European Alps or the chinook of the American Northwest. If so, the statement is quite accurate, since such winds do not cause throat and chest colds, but rather cardiac and circulatory disturbances.

Heart, lungs, liver, spleen, and kidneys are directly connected with the seasons and can therefore be affected by winds. Again, the warm foehn wind must be considered, which may also cause dyspnoea (shortness of breath), as well as irritability and depression. In persons with an acute cardiac disorder, foehns are also known to impede the discharge of urine.

The spleen, as befits such an elusive organ, pops up here and there throughout the system of correspondences, without any apparent motivation.

The Harmonious Balance Between the Different Flavors and the Organs

The heart, red, is in accordance with the pulse, controls the kidneys, and harmonizes with bitter flavors.

The lungs, white, are in accordance with the skin, control the heart, and harmonize with pungent flavors.

The liver, green, is in accordance with the muscles,* controls the lungs, and harmonizes with sour flavors.

The spleen, yellow, is in accordance with the flesh, controls the liver, and harmonizes with sweet flavors.

The kidneys, black, are in accordance with the bones, control the spleen, and harmonize with salty flavors.

The Aura of the Organs

The aura (health) condition of the five viscera may be determined from the colors of their corresponding "external organs."

* Was it perhaps known to the ancient Chinese that the liver—being a gland that generates metabolism—is an important support of the body's musculature?

Condition	Viscera	External organ in accordance with the viscera	Color of the external organ
inadequate	liver	muscles	green as young grass
	spleen	flesh	yellow-green as the fruits growing in copses
	kidneys	bones	black as coal
	heart	pulse	reddish-black as clotted blood
	lungs	skin	white as blanched and withered bones
flourishing	liver	muscles	green as the wings of the kingfisher
	spleen	flesh	yellow as a crab's belly
	kidneys	bones	black as a crow's wings
	heart	pulse	red as a cock's comb
	lungs	skin	white as pork fat

All colors must be fresh and shiny as silk.

What theoretical or practical value these assertions may possess, they certainly do not lack poetic truth in their description of colors. Granted that it seems quaint to imagine a clinical eye that perceives more than is dreamt of in our physiology, one fact is still indisputable: many an old practitioner—be he renowned professor or obscure country doctor—often makes better diagnoses from color, smell, and general appearance of the patient, than his colleagues do armed with microscope and textbook.

The Blood-Vessel System and the "Meridians" of Acupuncture

Medical trends in China, as those in the West, eventually led to over-specialization. This was to not a small degree the fault of the rigid doctrines of acupuncture, which was originally conceived as connected with the blood-vascular system. The minutest aspects of life and physical reactions had to be fitted into the theory of acupuncture (and its conflicting schools of thought), with the result that views became narrow but vague. Considering the highly sophisticated pulse theory, it seems odd that the theory of the blood vessels was largely a web of fantasy.

To cloud the issue further, later epochs divorced the

"meridians" of acupuncture entirely from any connection with the blood vessels. But the Chinese character for "meridian" continued to be translated as "artery," which fact, needless to say, caused much confusion in the West.

The Chinese must have been as perplexed by the blood vessels as the ancient Greek physicians were, who called the strong, gaping tubes "arteries," literally, "wind pipes." For when they came upon them in their autopsies—secret autopsies were obviously performed in China—and they cut into one of them, they may have found blood in it sometimes, but more frequently air.

The wall of an artery is elastic and keeps the shape of the vessel intact, even when it is empty. Since throughout the ancient world of East and West, the *pneuma*—air, breath—was an incomprehensible something (and still is, for that matter), it was only natural to assume that it was this *pneuma* that escaped from the dissected artery. This explains why some medical texts claim that blood emanates from certain acupuncture points, while *pneuma*, *Ch'i*, is released from others.

Blood and *Ch'i* are distributed within the *Yin* and *Yang* channels of the body as follows:

In *T'ai Yang* there is much blood and little *Ch'i*.
In *Shao Yang* there is little blood and much *Ch'i*.
In *Yang Ming* there is little blood and much *Ch'i*.
In *Shao Yin* there is little blood and much *Ch'i*.
In *Chüeh Yin* there is much blood and little *Ch'i*.
In *T'ai Yin* there is little blood and much *Ch'i*.

These channels constitute the basic meridians or "arteries"; beyond them, there are a number of other blood vessels, among them the eight "wondrous" vessels.

I. *Jen*   III. *Ch'ung*   V. *Yin Chi'ao*   VII. *Yin Wei*
II. *Tu*   IV. *Yang Chi'ao*   VI. *Yang Wei*   VIII. *Tai*

The Development of the Human Body

The following is a striking account of the various phases in the development of the male and the female body. If we substitute "reproductive gland" for the "kidney aura" of the man and the "*Jen* vessel" of the woman, the description could have been written today.

THE EIGHT-YEAR PHASES OF THE MALE BODY

At the age of eight, a boy's kidney aura grows strong, the hair grows thick and long, and his first teeth begin to fall out. At the age of two times eight, the kidney aura is developed to full vigor, and he begins to secrete semen. The more semen is emitted, the more desirous does the young man become of freeing himself of it. *Yin* and *Yang* (female and male) are in harmony throughout, and the man is able to beget children. At three times eight, the kidney aura is well balanced out; muscles and bones are powerful; the man has all his teeth and has reached his full height. At the age of four times eight, his muscles and bones are in splendid health and his flesh is firm and full. At five times eight, his kidney aura begins to decline, his hair begins to fall out, and his teeth begin to decay. At six times eight, his masculine vigor begins to slacken, his face becomes wrinkled, and his temples turn gray. At seven times eight, his liver aura begins to deteriorate, his muscles have lost their agility, and his semen emanates sparsely; the powers of the kidneys and his physical strength are dwindling rapidly. At eight times eight, he loses his teeth and his hair.

THE SEVEN-YEAR PHASES OF THE FEMALE BODY

At the age of seven, a girl's kidney aura grows strong, her baby teeth are beginning to fall out, and her hair grows long. At twice seven, she begins to menstruate, circulation starts in the *Jen* vessel, and her *Ch'ung* vessel grows strong. Menstruation is repeated regularly every month and the woman is capable of conceiving children. At three times seven years, her kidney aura has become steady, she has all her teeth, and her body is fully grown. At the age of four times seven, her muscles and bones are firm; her hair has grown to its full length; her whole body is at its blossoming best. At five times seven, the *Yang Ming* pulse ebbs, her face loses its moisture, and her hair begins to fall. At six times seven years, the pulses of all three *Yang* regions in the upper body wane, her face begins to wrinkle, and her hair turns gray. At the age of seven times seven, her *Jen* vessel runs dry and the *Ch'ung* vessel begins to harden. Menstruation occurs only rarely, the blood has ceased to circulate through her sexual organs, and she can no longer bear children.

V

CHINESE PATHOLOGY

The Cause of Diseases

Since it is the aim of this book to unveil hidden relationships and to whet the appetite for further exploration, some more specific points of the Chinese view of pathology must be offered here as guiding material.

As we know, it is a foregone conclusion for the Chinese that all diseases are caused by the disturbed harmony between *Yin* and *Yang*. Although at first glance this concept would seem to be a crass over-simplification of reality, it actually comes very close to modern thinking. For our twentieth-century physicians are once again convinced that a well-balanced disposition and the harmonious functioning of the nervous system are crucial requisites for a healthy body. If the so-called stress diseases are flourishing today, if high blood-pressure, peptic ulcers, and angina pectoris are tormenting the harried business executive, if we seem to be more sensitive to the moods and changes of the weather than our forefathers were, then it is probably partly due to the fact that our nerves are being impaired by the extremes of modern living. True enough, past eras had their own peculiar hazards, as has been pointed out by many observers. The French Revolution, the Thirty Years' War, the Norman Conquest were certainly no epochs of serene happiness for the people involved. Nevertheless, man's inner security seems to have been jolted out of balance more drastically during the past decades than ever before. Perhaps this is not so much the result of external catastrophes as the natural consequence of our loss of the "golden mean," our general withdrawal from the traditions of religion, mysticism, and philosophy.

But what matter? The fact remains that our nerves are on strike more frequently, and this phenomenon has incited scientific medicine to concern itself more intensely with the "*Yin* and *Yang*" within us. In doing so, modern scientists have arrived at some of the same conclusions as those put forth in the *Nei Ching* and other ancient texts: If the two complementing poles of life—stimulator and preserver, sympathetic and parasympathetic nervous system, consumer and storer, or whatever one chooses to call them—are not in coordination with one another, diseases will follow. And as pointed out at the beginning of this book, this basic principle of the bipolarity of life was verified anatomically when nerve fibers of the sympathetic system were discovered alongside those of the parasympathetic system, and vice versa. Once again, "within each *Yin* there is *Yang;* within each *Yang* there is *Yin.*"

Land Areas and Climates

Predominance in bringing about diseases is ascribed to climate and winds. Let the *Nei Ching* speak for itself:

	Heat—injures the heart.
The influence of the weather	Cold—injures the lungs.
on the five "internal" or-	Wind—injures the liver.
gans:	Humidity—injures the spleen.
	Dryness—injures the kidneys.

PECULIARITIES OF CLIMATE TO BE
CONSIDERED IN MAKING DIAGNOSES

In areas where the water is "light," there are many bald people, and goiters are frequent. In areas with "heavy" water, there are many paralytic people, or such that are suffering from dropsy. In areas with "pungent" water, malignant ulcers appear frequently. Where "bitter" water is found, many hunchbacks will be found as well.

CLIMATIC PECULIARITIES OF THE
CARDINAL POINTS

East is the region that engenders life (East—spring—sprouting are the correspondences). The animals of the sea thrive in that region and salt is abundant. The inhabitants of the East live mostly on fish and develop a constant craving for salt. Heavy consumption of fish injures the blood. (Salt makes one thirsty, and an unbalanced diet of fish alters the composition of the blood.) Thus, the inhabitants are of a darkish complexion, and they are frequently afflicted with abscesses and cancer. The most successful method of treatment for the diseases of these people is acupuncture with the flint-stone needle.

West is the region that produces metals and jade. Heaven and earth combine and are intent on gathering (West—autumn—harvesting). This region is sandy and strewn with rocks. Its inhabitants wear clothes made of wool and of straw, and they dwell mostly on hills. They are fond of good, rich food and are therefore fat and robust in appearance. Nothing can injure their physical bodies; diseases occur internally. Very potent medications are the treatment best suited for healing their illnesses.

North is the region of seclusion and storage (North—winter—preserving). This region is very mountainous, cold, and icy, and has frequent storms. Its people like to withdraw to lonesome, wild spots and nourish themselves on dairy products. The coldness is responsible for a multitude of diseases. The most appropriate means of curing them is moxibustion (cautery with the use of moxa, a preparation made from Chinese wormwood).

South is the region in which all the essences of life come to full bloom (South—summer—ripening). Beneath the surface of the earth, water flows, but the soil is languid. Therefore dew and mist collect above the earth. The inhabitants of the South love the color red and are fond of sour foods. They are susceptible to rheumatism and the gout. For these people, the most effective treatment is acupuncture with very fine needles.

The Middle is the region in which all the "ten thousand things" convene. This region is flat and humid. Its inhabitants receive their victuals from all directions and thus do not have to toil. Their illnesses are paralysis, catarrhs, and an inclination to high fevers. Gymnastics and massages are the best treatments.

The Winds

The east wind injures liver, throat, and neck.
The south wind injures heart, chest, and ribs.
The west wind injures lungs, shoulders, and back.
The north wind injures kidneys and hips.

As mentioned earlier, liver, heart, lungs, kidneys, and spleen live in direct interaction with the seasons and may be strongly affected by the winds. Throat, neck, chest, and ribs correlate only indirectly with the seasons and are therefore only slightly affected by the winds.

Winds are capable of generating a multitude of diseases. A cold wind causes a person's body-hair to stand up and closes the pores of the skin, so that fever heat accumulates in the body. An outbreak of perspiration, though, may bring rapid recovery. Cold winds may also create weakness, tumors, and pains. In such cases the illness should be dispersed with hot beverages, preferably soups, or through moxibustion.

If heat has not been administered early enough, the illness will advance into the lungs and cause pulmonary inflammation and coughing. If treatment is neglected further, the illness will extend into the liver and cause malfunction of the liver, pains in the ribs, and vomiting. Unless a cure can be attained through acupuncture at the ear-point, the illness will now penetrate into the spleen. This "wind-entry" into the spleen will bring about exhaustion, heat in the abdomen, cardiac disturbances, and jaundice. If at this point the disease cannot be expelled by medication or baths, it will advance into the kidneys, and this will manifest itself by the discharge of a whitish secretion.

This illness is also named the "worm disease," since flesh and body fat deteriorate as though chewed up by worms. If no medicaments can ameliorate the patient's condition, the disease will proceed to the heart. The muscles and arteries will tense up, which will lead to spasms. Now the only and very last resort is cautery with the use of moxa. And if that should prove unsuccessful, death will occur after the tenth day. For the kidneys have driven the disease into the heart; and the heart sends it back into the lungs, where fever heat will spread until three days later the patient is dead.

"Wind-entry" directly into the organs may germinate the following afflictions.

Wind entering the lungs: Respiratory difficulties and coughing, which are especially severe at night.

Wind entering the heart: Difficulties in speaking, lapses of memory, dry and chapped lips.

Wind entering the kidneys: Strangury (painful, constricted discharge of urine), bloated face, lumbago and other backaches after long periods of standing. All three maladies are accompanied by chills and sudden outbursts of perspiration.

Aside from the winds, over-exertion may be injurious to the body.

Prolonged straining of the eyes is harmful to the blood and the heart.
Prolonged lying in bed is harmful to the respiration and the lungs.*
Prolonged sitting is harmful to flesh and spine.
Prolonged standing is harmful to bones and kidneys.
Prolonged walking is harmful to muscles and liver.

Diagnoses According to Old Textbooks

The pulse theory was evidently the most highly developed diagnostic method in China. Naturally, this doctrine must also be stripped of much of its mystic adornment; but there is no doubt that, backed by adequate practice and rational judgment, pulse-reading could be used to better advantage today than it is. Several European physicians who have explored and applied the Chinese pulse theory maintain that they were able to make startling diagnoses which were subsequently verified by clinical tests. This intricate Chinese pulse system may not seem so unrealistic if we remember that a carefully observed pulse will yield more valuable information to the experienced heart specialist than to an untrained general practitioner.

In keeping with the strict tenets of the correspondences, the patient's coloring has to be considered for an effective diagnosis. Perhaps also this theory, if explored further, would reveal some worthwhile aspects that our technical laboratories may be concealing.

The condition of the tongue was another diagnostic aid to the Chinese physician, who was often not permitted to examine his patient in our Western sense, and who at times may not even have been aware of the identity of the person under his professional care. Like the rest of the body, the tongue was divided into definite sections, from whose appearance the symptoms of particular diseases could be read.

* Today's doctors discourage prolonged bed-rest, especially in older people, to prevent pneumonia.

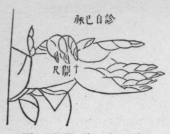

脉自已診

尺關寸

脉人他診

寸關尺

Fig. 37. Feeling the pulse with one's own hand.

Fig. 38. Pulse-taking by a physician.

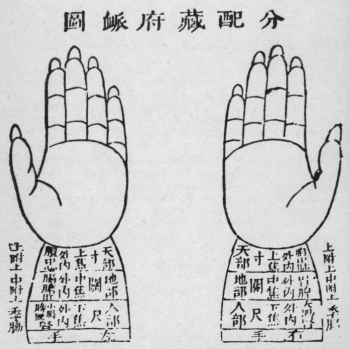

圖脈府藏配分

Fig. 39. The exact spots to touch when feeling the pulses.

Diagnoses Based on Pulse-Readings

If a modern physician wants to examine the condition of the wall of the artery, he feels the patient's pulse with his index, middle, and ring fingers. Just so does the Chinese physician of the traditional school place his fingers on the radial artery (artery in the forearm). However, Chinese doctors make a distinction between feeling one's own pulse and that of a patient. These differences are best illustrated in figures 37 to 39, although one cannot help but wonder at those overly long fingernails; granted that they were extremely elegant, but they must have presented a certain difficulty in feeling the pulse!

According to Chinese belief, there are many individual pulse types, all of which are somehow grouped in three main sections and are to be felt with the three fingers. The index finger feels the ts'un or "inch" pulse (ts'un—one inch); the middle finger feels the kuan or "passage" pulse (kuan—"passage," "path"); and the ring finger feels the ch'ih or "cubit" pulse (ch'ih—one cubit).

These three main pulse groups are believed to reveal different physical conditions in left and right wrist. Moreover, each of the three double sections is divided into two major pulse groups: the "external, superficial" pulse, called the piao pulse, of which there are seven, and the "sunken, hidden, internal" pulse, called the li pulse, of which there are eight in the group.

To make this complex system quite clear to the students, some textbooks augment the description of the individual pulse types with diagrams, such as those shown in figures 41 to 46. The ideographs for the three main sections are easily discernible at the center of each circle.

The pulse in general is considered the storehouse of the blood. When the pulse strokes are long and deliberate (what today might be termed a strong pulse), then the aura (life-impulse) is in good health. When the pulse beats are short, the aura is impaired. When the strokes are hurried, then they indicate that the heart is injured. When the pulse beats are large and full, a grave illness is about to develop.

When the pulse beat is abundant, then the body is distended. When pulsation is erratic and tangled as weed, then the aura is wilting. When it is tender, tremulous, and skips beats now and then, very little life-impulse is left. When the pulse strokes are frail, wavering to and fro, and limping, there will be pains in the heart (cardiac pains are frequent with an irregular, unrhythmic pulse, as is well known today).

As said above, the pulse beats of each hand have to be evaluated differently, because each section registers the condition of certain parts of the body.

PULSES AND THEIR CORRESPONDING ORGANS

Pulse Section	Hand	Organ or Part of Body
Ts'un	right	lungs, chest, gall bladder
	left	mediastinal viscera (heart, etc.)
Kuan	right	stomach, spleen
	left	liver, diaphragm
Ch'ih	right	kidney, abdominal cavity, large intestine
	left	kidney, abdominal cavity, small intestine

PULSE CHARACTERISTICS FOR THE

INDIVIDUAL ORGANS

The heart pulse should be like the ringing sound of a sickle: rich at first, then trailing off.

The spleen pulse should alternate in a regular rhythm.

The lung pulse should flow evenly and softly, like hair or feathers blowing in the wind.

The kidney pulse should beat with deep and resounding strokes, like a stone hitting the ground.

The liver pulse should sound mellow as the string of a musical instrument.

It is of course quite understandable when the modern technician, who observes the patient's pulse with sphygmograph, amplifier, and Braun tube, shows little patience with the claim that the pulsation is "mellow as the string of a musical instrument" or that it "flows softly, like hair blowing in the wind." But by the same token it must be doubted whether his machines would ever be sensitive enough to feel such subtle differences. Perhaps such differences do not exist, but it is likely that the last word has not been spoken on the subject.

THE SEVEN "PIAO" PULSES AND THE

EIGHT "LI" PULSES

How very "palpable" these individual pulse types were to the Chinese is quite apparent from all medical textbooks.

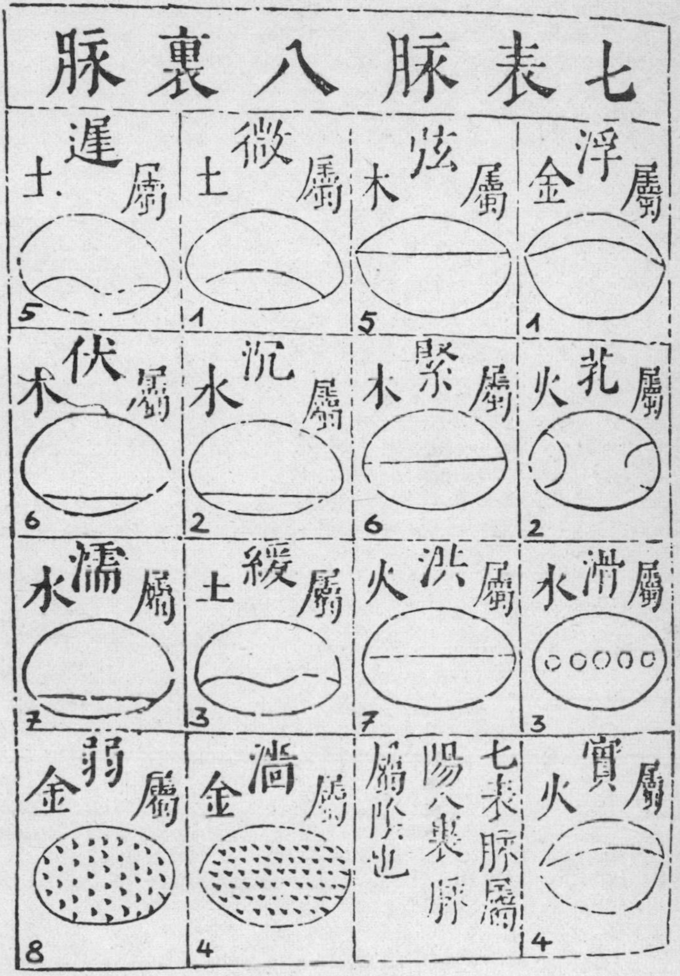

Fig. 40. An ideogrammatic representation of the pulse types.

Some of the Chinese "pulse curves" might almost be favorably compared to the writings of the modern pulsimeter.

The "external" *piao* pulses and the "internal" *li* pulses are rather ingeniously transmitted in the illustrations in figure 40. The lines within the ovals symbolize the characters of the individual pulse types. The numbers in the squares correspond to the numbers of the descriptive text following below. In figure 40, the numbers are to be read from top to bottom, starting in the upper right-hand corner.

The seven piao *pulses ("superficial" pulses)*

1. Floating; gliding like a fish or like a piece of wood in the water.
2. Feeble and empty; it feels like an onion stalk that is empty in the middle and firm on both sides.
3. Slippery; like a string of pearls gliding through one's fingers.
4. Full and long.
5. Stretched like the string of a lute.
6. Tight; as if a rope were being twisted firmly.
7. Large; flowing majestically.

The eight li *pulses ("sunken" pulses)*

1. Unassuming; a small, faint pulse, hidden, and dying away at intervals.
2. Sunk deeply inside; like a pebble thrown into the water (the "weak, small" pulse of today?).
3. Scattered, slow; like a willow dancing in the spring breeze.
4. Wavering to and fro, limping; it comes up slowly, fades away, or stops short, like a knife shaving bamboo, or like raindrops plopping into sand.
5. Slow, hesitant; three beats to one cycle of respiration (i.e., approximately forty-eight beats per minute).
6. Crouched, fallen; even when applying pressure, this pulse is difficult to feel.
7. Timidly hidden and tender.
8. Frail, plaint, gliding; extremely weak.

GENERAL GUIDING RULES FOR THE DIAGNOSIS FROM THE "PIAO" AND "LI" PULSES WITHIN EACH OF THE THREE SECTIONS

The following illnesses manifest themselves in the seven *piao* pulses:

a) Within *ts'un:*

1. Pains and heat in the middle region of the body and in the head.
2. Accumulation of blood in the chest.
3. Belching and vomiting.
4. Insufferable heat within the thorax.
5. Severe thoracic pains.
6. Headaches.
7. Heat in the chest.

b) Within *kuan:*

1. Hollow feeling in the stomach; swollen abdomen.
2. Intestinal ulcers.
3. Coldness in the stomach; indigestion.
4. Pains in the region of the lower ribs.
5. Coldness in the stomach.
6. Lumbar pains; difficulty in moving about.
7. Repeated attacks of nausea.

c) Within *ch'ih:*

1. Wind in the lungs; constipation; desiccated bowels.
2. Depletion of the kidneys; blood in the urine.
3. Coldness in the abdomen.
4. Bloated belly; strangury (painful and difficult urine discharge).
5. Accumulation of fluid in the abdomen.
6. Pains in navel and belly.
7. Reddish and scalding urine discharge; aches in the feet.

The following illnesses manifest themselves in the eight *li* pulses:

a) Within *ts'un:*

1. Accumulation of air in thorax and head.
2. Mucus in the chest.
3. Neuralgias.
4. Queasy stomach.
5. Coldness above the heart.
6. Accumulation of air in the chest.
7. Excessive perspiration of the feet.
8. Emptiness in *Yang Tao;* exhaustion.

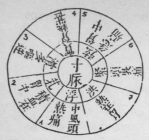

Fig. 41. The 7 *piao* pulses within the *ts'un* section.

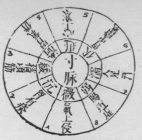

Fig. 44. The 8 *li* pulses within the *ts'un* section.

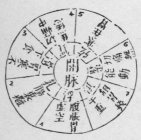

Fig. 45. The 8 *li* pulses within the *kuan* section.

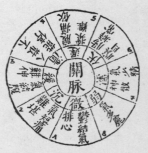

Fig. 42. The 7 *piao* pulses within the *kuan* section.

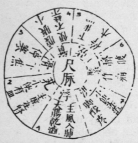

Fig. 43. The 7 *piao* pulses within the *ch'ih* section.

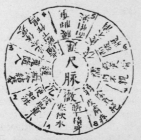

Fig. 46. The 8 *li* pulses within the *ch'ih* section.

b) Within *kuan:*

1. Anxiety.
2. Short and stinging breath.
3. Abdominal gases; difficulty in standing erect.
4. Restlessness; indecisiveness.
5. Pains in abdomen; difficulty swallowing.
6. Weakened bowels; eyes closing involuntarily and repeatedly.
7. Body stamina very low; absent-mindedness.
8. Respiratory difficulties; panting.

c) Within *ch'ih:*

1. Coldness below the navel; continual feeling of thirst.
2. Feeling of heaviness in waist region and legs; thickening of the urine.
3. Constipation; feeling of coldness; dreams of being persecuted.
4. Oppressive feeling of coldness in body and limbs; murmurs below the navel.
5. Feeling of heaviness and cold in lumbar area and legs.
6. Dyspepsia; diarrhea.
7. Insufferable feeling of coldness, and of flesh and bones being disconnected.
8. Stoppage of the *Yin*-breath; stiffness; aching skin.

GUIDING PRINCIPLES FOR FAVORABLE AND UNFAVORABLE PULSES DURING THE FOUR SEASONS

The spring pulse is the liver pulse. The cardinal point corresponding to spring is the East, the correlated element, wood. The "ten thousand things" begin to germinate and develop. The pulse should come up easily but firmly and should swell like the sound of a lute string. When the strokes are too full and too vigorous, an external disease is befalling the patient; when the strokes are timid and have but little volume, an internal disease is setting in. If the pulse is overly abundant, the corresponding disease will incline the patient toward anger, mental derangement, and finally madness. A flaccid pulse-beat indicates pains in chest and ribs.

The summer pulse is the heart pulse. The cardinal point corresponding to summer is the South, the correlated element, fire. All "ten thousand things" are now blossoming in full splendor. The beat of the summer pulse should emerge amply and move away gently, like the swinging cut of a sickle. When the strokes are ample in going as well as coming, then an external disease is arising. When they are gentle in coming but ample in moving away, an internal disease has set in. When the pulse is overly abundant, the corresponding disease will cause heat within the body; the skin will hurt and become clammy. A frail pulse will make the patient cross and restless. Coughing with expectoration will result, and the impulse of life will drift away.

The autumn pulse is the pulse of the lungs. The cardinal point corresponding to autumn is the West, the correlated element, metal. The "ten thousand things" are now fully ripened and are waiting to be harvested. The pulse should come up lightly and empty, and should be swift in leaving. When the strokes of the autumn pulse come up roughly, are firm in the middle and hollow on both sides, an external disease is taking hold; when the strokes are rough but feeble, then they denote an internal disease. When the pulse is overly abundant, the corresponding disease will cause shortness of breath and backaches, and will make the patient irritable and discontented. A weak pulse denotes shortness of breath accompanied by the coughing of blood (hemoptysis).

The winter pulse is the pulse of the kidneys. The cardinal point corresponding to winter is the North, the correlated element, water. The "ten thousand things" are now securely stored, and the pulse beats should thus be deep and resolute. When the stroke comes up hard, like hitting a stone, an external disease is setting in. When the pulse withdraws with a run of quick beats, an internal disease is spreading. An opulent pulse denotes pains in the spine, respiratory difficulties, and an unwillingness to speak. When the winter pulse is too fragile, the corresponding illness will create a feeling of excessive hunger, flatulence in the belly, and difficulty in urinating.

The spleen, this eccentric organ of all organs, influences the other organs from its isolated position. Its element is earth. When the condition of the spleen is healthy and sound, then it does not manifest itself at all in any way. But when the spleen pulse rushes like cascading water, an external disease is arising; when it is like the pecking of a bird's beak, an internal disease has befallen the patient. When the pulse is too profuse, the corresponding illness will render the patient incapable of lifting his limbs. When the pulse is too weak, then the corresponding illness causes agony, because the patient's nine orifices are not interacting harmoniously.

THE PULSE OF EPILEPTICS

The pulse indicating the most favorable prognosis for an epileptic is a slow pulse, floating like a piece of wood on the water. When the pulse becomes full and vigorous and begins to accelerate, the patient will clamp his teeth, and foam will appear at his mouth. When his pulse beats are twisted like a piece of rope and are full, vigorous and accelerated at the same time, then the patient will flail about wildly, and oily beads of perspiration will soon cover his body. When in addition the patient's complexion changes into a bluish pallor, his condition is critical (a statement that coincides with modern observations).

THE PULSE OF PREGNANT WOMEN

When the pulse of the woman's left wrist is hurried, without slowing down or dissolving gradually, she will give birth to a boy. When the pulse of her right wrist shows these characteristics, a girl may be expected.

It occurs frequently that a woman is not aware of her condition. But if the *ts'un* pulse is delicate and concealed, the *kuan* pulse slippery, and the *ch'ih* pulse accelerated, a pregnancy may be diagnosed with fair certainty.

PULSE CHARACTERISTICS FORETELLING DEATH

When the liver pulse ceases, internal and external agitation will follow, whereupon the patient will have the sensation of being threatened by a falling sword, or of a lute string being forced down hard. His face will turn a greenish-white and will lose its glow; his body-hair breaks, and death is inevitable.

When the heart pulse loses its vigor but pops incessantly like the seeds of a water lily, then the face will turn a reddish-black and lose its glow; the body-hair will break, and death is imminent.

When the kidney pulse beats jerkily as though a finger were snapping against a stone and bouncing back, the patient's complexion will turn yellow-black and lose its glow; his body-hair breaks, and death is imminent.

When the lung pulse ceases to beat daintily and lightly like feathers or hairs blowing in the wind, the patient's skin becomes a hectic white-red and loses its glow; his body-hair will break and death is imminent.

When the spleen pulse ceases to beat in its alternating rhythm of quick and slow strokes, the patient's face will turn yellowish-green and lose its glow; the body-hair will break, and death is imminent.

These are the irrevocable heralds of death, making themselves known in the pulses of the five viscera; no cure in the whole world can be of any further help.

PULSES AND COLORS

For a "more precise" examination, the Chinese physician also takes into account the colors corresponding to the five organs. Only when they are observed in conjunction with the pulses can a complete picture of the illness be obtained.

When a patient's coloring is red and his breath forceful, then too much air has collected in the heart. It is unadvisable to consume food during that period (gastric gases). This illness is called "inadequacy of the heart." It is caused by outer influences and emotional disturbances which penetrate into the heart and deplete it of its life-force. (The same causes are cited today for disturbances of the cardiovascular system—the "executive's disease.")

When a patient's coloring is white, when his breath flows but faintly, when the *piao* pulse is empty and the *li* pulse full, then the patient has suffered a frightening shock. Air has accumulated in the chest; hence the breath is empty and fleeting. This illness is called "distension and rupture of the lung cells" (pulmonary emphysema?). It is caused by fever-heat and cold.

When the patient's coloring is green and the pulse strokes in both wrists are long, then air has collected in the heart and at the lower ribs. This illness is called "weakness of the liver" and is caused by chill, dampness, and cold feet.

When the patient's coloring is yellow and the pulse beats are long-drawn, hollow, and exhausted, then air and gases have collected in the abdomen. This illness is called "flatulence"; women, too, may be seized by it. It develops when a person perspires in the four limbs and is subsequently exposed to drafty winds.

When the patient's coloring is black and when the *piao* pulse is sturdy and large, air has collected in the pelvis. This illness is called "weak kidneys," and it is ofen caused by dampness around the abdomen. The patient should bathe in pure water, lie down, and rest.

Further Diagnostic Possibilities

DIAGNOSIS FROM THE TONGUE

Diagnosing a disease from the condition of the tongue is a realm all by itself. The Chinese doctor differentiates between more than one hundred varieties of tongue condition. Like all other parts of the body, the tongue, too, is related very closely to the viscera:

The middle of the tongue is correlated with the stomach.
The two sides of the tongue are correlated with the liver.
The root of the tongue is correlated with the kidneys.
The tip of the tongue is correlated with the heart.

As may be expected, the coloring of the tongue is as relevant to the diagnosis as is the tongue's overall condition and its fur.

DIAGNOSES BASED ON THE MOODS OF THE PATIENT

Persons suffering from liver ailments appear most perspicacious during the morning hours, are lively and animated toward sundown, and of tranquil mind at midnight.

Persons with cardiac illnesses are at their most perspicacious around noonday, lively and animated at midnight, and tranquil in the early morning.

Patients with diseases of the spleen appear most perspicacious just after sundown, lively and animated at sunrise, and are tranquil during the afternoon.

Persons suffering from pulmonary diseases are perspicacious just before sundown, are lively and animated at noon, and are tranquil at midnight.

Patients with kidney diseases are most perspicacious at midnight, lively and animated during the last days of all four seasons, and are at their most tranquil before sundown.

OTHER SYMPTOMS DENOTING DISEASED ORGANS

Afflicted Organ	Symptoms
Lungs	Coughing; short-windedness; asthma; bronchitis; headache; nausea; hot palms; restlessness; nervous tension.
Spleen	Stomach ache, indigestion or diarrhea; heavy body; limbs as though paralyzed;

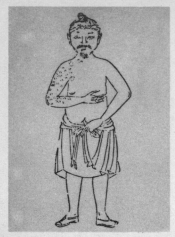

Fig. 47. *Herpes zoster?*

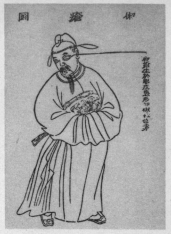

Fig. 48. Granular inflammation of the conjunctiva (trachoma?).

Fig. 49. "Rash like the eggs of the silk moth."

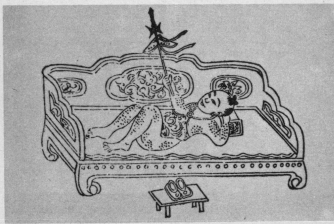

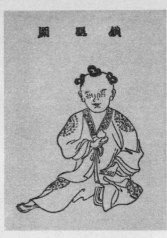

Fig. 50. Conjunctivitis.

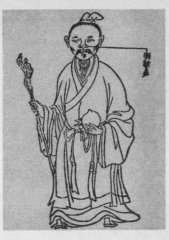

Fig. 51. An alcoholic's nose.

Fig. 52. "The broken bridge."

Fig. 53. Bandage for knee injuries.

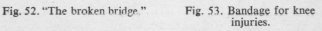

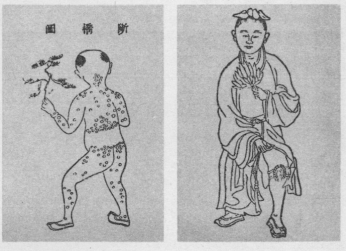

the root of the tongue aches; pains in the hollow of the knee; oppressive palpitation of the heart; nervousness combined with listlessness; difficulty in moving the big toes.

Large Intestine   Toothaches; headache; reddened eyes; dry palate; inflamed throat; disorder in the digestive tract; numb feeling in first and second fingers.

Kidneys   Complexion black as coal; respiratory difficulties; swollen throat; hot feeling in mouth; dry tongue; pains in the heart, the back, and in the abdomen; hot, tired feet; fear of people; anxieties; restlessness.

Bladder   Headache; stiff neck; pains in back and lumbago; difficulty in bending; expectoration of blood; persistent cold in the nose; scalding of the bladder; eyes yellow and watery; difficulty in moving the little finger.

DIAGNOSES BASED ON PERSPIRATION

After a copious meal with plenty of beverages, perspiration will make its appearance through the stomach.

After a sudden shock of terror, the essence of life is defeated; perspiration will be generated from the heart.

After hauling a heavy burden over a long distance, perspiration will emanate from the kidneys.

After a strenuous task requiring great physical strength, perspiration will emerge from the spleen.

After a walk in undue haste combined with feelings of anxiety, perspiration will originate in the liver.

Curiosities from Old Medical Textbooks
Describing Diseases

From early times in Chinese medical history, illustrations have always accompanied descriptions of diseases as adjuncts to the data on pulses, colors, aura-conditions, perspiration, and other symptoms. Such drawings were meant to enlighten the student on particular aspects of the illness, and indeed they do. However, there are some instances where the diagrams defy proper interpretation. Even with the help of Chinese physicians, the authors were not always able to find exact modern counterparts to the Chinese denominations of the diseases portrayed in those drawings. But it seems more than justified to assume that figure 47 demonstrates a case of *herpes zoster* (inflammatory affection of the skin on one side of the body following the course of a nerve). An eye disease (trachoma?) in an adult person, and another one (conjunctivitis?) in a child, are evidently depicted in figures 48 and 50 respectively, while the patient's visage in figure 51 obviously betrays the bliss of the alcoholic state; the beauty of his sottish nose can hardly be misinterpreted.

Figure 54—as the medical reader probably suspects— illustrates various types of hemorrhoids. They are excellently observed; and it might be added that it must have been a trying task—even for the patience of a Chinese—to create such a minute schematization of hemorrhoidal forms. It will probably no longer surprise anyone to learn that the shapes of hemorrhoids were employed in diagnosing other diseases also.

THE VARIOUS TYPES OF HEMORRHOIDS

The following list describes the hemorrhoidal forms pictured in figure 54. The pictures are to be read from top to bottom, the columns taken in the order of the roman numerals.

I   1. (Illegible on the print)
     2. The flesh of a mussel
     3. A hanging pearl
     4. Enclosure of an intestine
     5. A chestnut
     6. A walnut

II   1. Seeds of the lotus flower
     2. Prolapse of the rectum
     3. Anchor of an intestine
     4. A chicken heart
     5. A cow's udder
     6. Tail of a rat

III 1. Clots of blood
     2. Support for the bowels
     3. Internal hemorrhoids
     4. Cherries

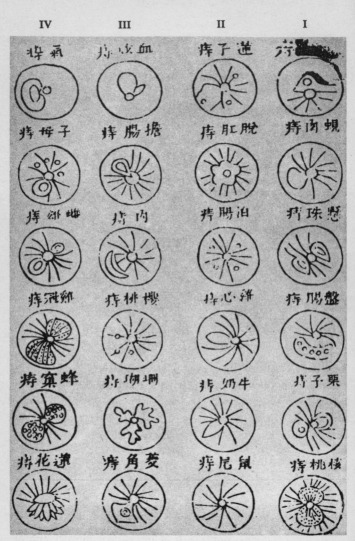

Fig. 54. Various types of hemorrhoids.

5. Protecting walls of a fortress
6. An ocean plant

IV 1. Air bubbles
    2. Sons with their mother
    3. Hermaphrodite
    4. A cock's comb
    5. A honeycomb
    6. Lotus flower

BREAST CANCER AND MALARIA

In a recently published analysis of Chinese medical ideograms and characters, Dr. Gottfried Schramm makes the following interesting observation: "A red and white discharge [of urine] was known [to the Chinese] from early times, as were descriptions of breast cancer." In one of Dr. Franz Hübotter's translations we find these words: "The disease begins with a knot in the breast, the size of a bean, and gradually swells to the size of an egg. After seven or eight months it perforates. When it has perforated, it is very difficult to cure." This Chinese statement can hold its own against any description of breast cancer in modern surgical textbooks.

Very revealing also are the various names by which malaria was known in different provinces. Here is the list as it appears in Dr. Schramm's work:

Coldness entering the body	Heat entering the body
The chill-disease	Quilt over skin
To get the shivers	Tingling in fingertips
To catch small chickens	Devil's disease
Disease of the five devils	Fever-chill
The veritable illness	The irresistible malaria
The venerable old gentleman	Dumpling in the belly
The daily disease	Three days
Once in three days	The one hundred days disease
The fluctuating days	
The one forever recurring	Three fever attacks within two days

Each one of these descriptive phrases discloses a good deal of poignant observation, both of the patient himself and of the course of the disease. Schramm, for example, suggests that the expression "dumpling in the belly" refers to the swelling of the spleen that always accompanies severe attacks of malaria.

Nor did the Old Chinese stray too far from reality when they assumed that eels were the cause of malaria. (At certain periods in history, veritable eel-hunts were conducted in order to extirpate the pestilential disease.) Where is the larva of the anopheles mosquito hatched if not in the regions that are half land and half water and that are also the habitat of eels?

Equally well known in Old China was blackwater fever, a complication of malaria resulting especially from overdoses of quinine.

VI

CHINESE TREATMENT METHODS

MRS. LI LIU IS EXPECTING

Happy, excited, and a trifle nervous, Mrs. Li Liu was looking forward to her important moment. She was expecting her first child and she most ardently hoped for a boy. Fortunately, the astrologer who had compared her own and her husband's horoscopes before their engagement had prophesied a prevailingly male progeny.

Throughout the nine months, Mrs. Li Liu had observed all the prescribed instructions conscientiously and could thus hope to give birth to a healthy child. When upon awaking she had discovered that she had slept on one side only for a long time, she had immediately turned over on the other, so that the baby would develop evenly. When it was absolutely necessary that she bend down, she would do so with the greatest circumspection. In like manner, she had avoided prolonged standing and had evaded every kind of quarrel, every ugly sight, and every discordant sound. She had abstained completely from fatty foods, not to mention spicy dishes. And she had not let a day go by without making her votive offering to Kuan Yin, so that the goddess might deliver a soul unto the new-born.

Mrs. Li Liu could now cast aside all fears and apprehensions. Moreover, her mother-in-law and her sister-in-law were all convinced that she would be delivered of a boy; for was not her belly shaped like a kettle, round and full at the bottom and slimming toward the top? Aye—and that was an infallible sign of the birth of a male offspring.

Kuan Yin, the Goddess of Fertility

Kuan Yin, "she who looks down and heeds the suppliant cries of man," is worshiped as the goddess of fertility and motherly love. In contrast to most other deities, she is not inaccessible and awe-inspiring, but merciful, compassionate, and sympathetic to human suffering. She is therefore ardently loved and admired.

As legend has it, she has experienced the life of an ordinary mortal, with all its perils and vicissitudes, which naturally serves to weave an even tighter bond between the goddess and her worshipers. True to her nature, she leaves no entreaty unanswered; she rescues the sailor from a shipwreck and the traveler who is lost in foreign lands; she also provides for the sick and the poor; and, last but not least, she saves the guilt-ridden by lifting all traces of evil thoughts from their minds. When one prays to her, an aura of peace and balm will arise inside one's heart, and all earthly sorrows will drift away.

But Kuan Yin's special attention is reserved for the women who beseech her to bless them with children. For she knows well the sorrows of those who are denied such a blessing.

Numberless representations of Kuan Yin are in existence. Up to the twelfth century, she was often pictured with masculine instead of feminine features. Since then, however, her image appears most frequently clad in a long, flowing white robe, denoting her purity; sometimes she is sitting on a throne of lotus blossoms; at other times she is standing on a tall rock, a child in her arms. Other sources show her riding a dragon while holding the twig of a willow in one hand and a bowl filled with the dew of immortality in the other. Occasionally she is also represented as the thousand-armed goddess, showering mercy and consolation upon mankind.

Chinese Pediatrics

The immense over-population under which China has always suffered (today's estimate is about 690 million Chinese) has at various times in history resulted in the practice of infanticide. The newly born babies were either drowned or were suffocated by spreading over their faces a piece of paper soaked in vinegar.

To make sure that the child would develop a slender head, which was considered extremely noble, mothers would let babies sleep on their sides only. This custom was still practiced at the beginning of the Ch'ing Dynasty (1644), but it dates back to about 2200 B.C., when it had been a sign of the utmost beauty to have a wide chin and a long head slimming to a point at the crown. This coveted head-shape was attained by methods more or less dangerous and similar to those encountered even today among some African tribes. It is owing solely to the unbelievable adaptability of the human organism that such experiments do not always have a fatal ending.

Cow's milk and goat's milk were spurned in China as nourishment for babies. Mothers and wet-nurses would often breast-feed their infants for as long as four or five years. This disdain for goat's milk will not seem so implausible when we remember that a type of nutritional anemia occurs frequently in areas where infants are maintained chiefly on a goat's milk diet.

Vaccination as a prophylaxis for smallpox was known in China at a very early time. The dreaded plague that slaughtered thousands of children was known by the euphemistic name "budding of blossoms." A similar illness was called "a rash like the eggs of the silk moth" (see figure 49). From an equally early date stems the recognition that a second smallpox infection in one person is extremely rare. At that time, of course, Chinese physicians were not yet familiar with the use of a killed or mitigated bacterium for vaccinating; instead, the child was inoculated with the fully active smallpox virus, thus being subjected to a true infection. To this end, the crust of a pustula from a smallpox patient was pulverized and then blown into the child's nose by means of a thin tube. Since the body of a healthy child so treated would have enough natural resistance, those early physicians were justified to some extent in expecting the disease to take a rather mild course, the more so since for such a "vaccine" only the scabs of very light pox cases were used; it is again surprising how correct and very "modern" that approach was.

Other sources recommended wrapping the child in robes that had been smeared with pus from mild smallpox cases in order to expose the child to a moderate infection of the disease. This method, incidentally, was also practiced very early in India. An even more intriguing Indian procedure is the following one: The skin was scratched with a sharp instrument, and into the scratch wound was rubbed the suppuration of a pox pustula—which is, of course, almost our modern procedure, except that non-virulent vaccine lymph has replaced the pustular suppuration.

LI FANG AND HIS FINAL EXAM

The young Li Fang lay in his bed and sighed. Not a wink had he been able to sleep last night, for a horrible fear had haunted him during all those hours of darkness: the fear that he would fail the forthcoming final examination. Yes, he had excelled at the oral exam only the day before and, yes, he had answered without hesitation all questions put before him from the *Nei Ching* and the *Pen Ts'ao*, as well as those from the other fine works of medicine. And it was true that the jury of professors had been well satisfied with the prescriptions for medicines that he had named for the various diseases. Yet, in a few short hours he would have to demonstrate his skill in the most difficult and most crucial subject: Acupuncture.

Li Fang rose from his bed, worried and apprehensive, clad himself carefully in his very best garments, as custom demanded, and set out on his way to the examination hall. Serious and probing were the looks on the professors' faces when Li Fang entered the auditorium. With his heart pounding in his throat, he watched the attendant as the latter walked to the table and placed on it that figure of wood that presently was to decide his fate.

He had studied incessantly during the past months until he knew all 365 acupuncture points by heart and was able to choose the correct point each time with a swift, decisive thrust of the needle. But now that he was actually faced with that wooden statue—which had been filled with water and coated with a layer of wax for the test—his self-confidence seemed to evaporate. His eyes fixed on the statue as though it were an evil ghost; he hardly heard it when his name was called. He was ordered to step up to the table.

Before he could regain his composure, the most honorable professor who was feared by all students as especially relentless had fired the first question at him: "How do you treat a patient when his kidney aura is weaknened, when the heart-section of his tongue denotes a like weakness of the corresponding organ, and when his *ts'un* pulse is taut like the string of a musical instrument?"

The candidate pulled himself together and named a certain acupuncture spot. With an obviously pleased nod, the examiner invited Li Fang to try the puncture at the place he had indicated.

Mustering up all his courage, the young doctor-to-be grabbed the needle, paused for a second in concentration, and jabbed it into the wax, and—his heart jumped with joy —at once the water gushed forth from the tiny hole. The first question had been answered correctly! Encouraged by this success, he was now able to solve all the other problems to the entire satisfaction of the professors.

Li Fang passed the examination and thus became a doctor of medicine and an acupuncture specialist.

Acupuncture and Modern Therapies

In 1893, the British neurologist Sir Henry Head (1861–1940) published a discovery which was to assure him a lasting name in medical textbooks, although initially it aroused but little attention. Head had observed that patients suffering from gall bladder or renal attacks did not necessarily have pains in the afflicted organs, but that their pains were referred to certain, and clearly definable, areas of the skin. These "Head's zones," as they have come to be called in medical science, have provided the progressive physician of our era with a score of new treatment possibilities. Even a simple massage or diathermy on these specific skin areas has proved of surprisingly beneficial effect. Lately, the field of therapeutic anesthesia has made notable use of the theory underlying Head's zones. The term "therapeutic anesthesia" is a direct translation of the German *Heilanästhesie* and is not included in American medical terminology. The therapy as such is practiced in America and includes such methods as nerve-blocking by the injection of a local anesthetic for the relief of somatic or visceral pains, and the very recently developed method of intravenous anesthesia with a local anesthesia for the same purpose (see Dr. Huneke's researches, described below).

It must be added in all fairness that Head was not the first to discover such cutaneous zones. As early as 1834, the Swedish hygienist Pehr Henrik Ling (1776–1839) had perceived the same phenomenon; and shortly thereafter, but unrelated to Ling's reports, the brothers W. and D. Griffin, physicians in America, published their observations on referred pain in certain zones associated with diseases of the viscera.

Another of Head's forerunners was the homeopathist Dr. Weihe, who issued the results of his investigations in 1883. Weihe professed to have discovered 195 points in close affinity with the viscera—quite similar to acupuncture points. Although translations of Chinese treatises on acupuncture were available at the time, Dr. Weihe appears to have had no knowledge of them. It is therefore remarkable that many of Weihe's points correspond to the points mentioned in the Chinese texts.

Weihe's disclosures later prompted some of his colleagues to come to their own elaborate conclusions about a connection between acupuncture and homeopathy. But it certainly takes an emphatic believer in the homeopathic school to accept all of Weihe's and his followers' assumptions without objection.

For a period of several years, the IG Farben concern in Germany awarded a grant to a physician in the field of neuropathology, allowing him to experiment with a combination of Novocain and caffeine, in order to obtain an anesthetic for curative purposes. At the time, this physician—the now renowned Dr. Huneke of Düsseldorf—was considered something of an eccentric and dreamer. But as Dr. Huneke himself relates, the director of the Pharmaceutical Department pronounced: "What does it matter to IG Farben at this point whether Huneke is a crackpot or not? But what if he should turn out to be right? We would never be able to live down the shame for having overlooked him."

What had started Dr. Huneke on his pursuit was the accidental discovery that he was able to cure an obstinate migraine in one of his patients by an intravenous injection of Novocain, which had been reserved for local anesthesia. With that incident alone, however, Huneke had not yet reached the crux of therapeutic anesthesia. Another accident was to advance him further. During the administering of an intravenous injection, the needle slid off the vein and the injection went in beside the vein, i.e., paravenously, whereupon his patient was rid of her pains instantly, as though touched by a magic wand. Huneke recalls: "At that moment, the whole structure of our hard-earned medical concepts crumbled to pieces."

The structure of twentieth-century medical concepts has been, and is still being, shaken by many more new discoveries about fundamentals. Research laboratories throughout the world can attest to this.

More than a few scholars have come to acknowledge the close similarity between therapeutic anesthesia and the more than 2,000-year-old therapy of acupuncture, overgrown though the latter may be with a tangled mass of imagery and superstition.

Admittedly, the relationship is often rather loose and will not always withstand close scrutiny. One fact, though, seems certain: with the practice of any branch of therapeutic anesthesia we are venturing into the region of the complex interplay of the nerves to an extent that we cannot yet fully realize. In fact, nobody knows exactly how or why a method like the above-mentioned intravenous injection with a local anesthetic does work. Meanwhile, though, some stunning and undeniable cures have been achieved with it.

The same cure is sought after when the Chinese doctor inserts his sharp needle in the acupuncture point. As the teachings of acupuncture claim, each internal organ is in close affinity with its own definite spots, or points, on the skin. There are 365 in all, and they are distributed all over the body, including the head and limbs. The insertion of the needle in these respective points is said to exert either a stimulating or an equalizing effect, thereby reinstating order and harmonious balance within the disturbed collaboration of the nerves—or of *Yin* and *Yang*, as the Chinese have it. Most research scientists agree that in its deepest essence, this concept corresponds to the Western theory of the sympathetic and parasympathetic nervous system; only die-hard skeptics still refuse to acknowledge the curative results that have been attained in some cases by the mere insertion of a gold, silver, or steel needle. On the other hand, it seems only just to demand that the acupuncture fanatics concede the obvious fact that not every disease can be cured by this therapy.

Until the turn of this century, acupuncture was practiced solely in the oriental hemisphere and was completely unknown in other countries. Its application goes back to ancient times, although there were probably far fewer puncture points originally, as Professor K. Saller suggests. Like any other medical treatment method, acupuncture, too, has lived through its high and its low epochs.

While it had fallen into neglect around A.D. 600, it began to blossom again during the following T'ang Dynasty (618), the golden age of medicine, and gained wide popularity during the generally energetic and alert Sung Dynsty (960–1126). During the T'ang period an academic chair solely for the discipline of acupuncture was established. And it was during this epoch that the wooden figures became popular for student practice. For examinations, the figures were covered with wax in order to conceal the points of insertion from the candidates. In the years since, these wooden statues have become an indispensable aid and are still used today in the very same manner.

THE PURPOSE OF ACUPUNCTURE

Acupuncture is based on the following concept: Certain channels or ducts—now usually called meridians—extend internally (perhaps imbedded in the muscles) throughout the body in a fixed network. The 365 points on the skin are the spots where those meridians emerge on the surface. Since skin points, meridians, and viscera are interrelated, and since all of them naturally harbor the ebb and flow of *Yin* and *Yang,* a cure is believed possible by treating one of the cutaneous "outlet" points.

The insertion of needles into these strategic points is designed to diminish an "abundance" (excess) or to replenish a "deficiency," depending on the particular need of the diseased organ. It is assumed that the stagnated *pneuma* is drained, and young, fresh *pneuma* is substituted. Hence, the puncture points may also be considered the "gate-keepers" for their affected meridians and organs. But in certain cases the points may also function indirectly as gate-keepers for other meridians.

After the doctor has made a precise diagnosis based on the syndromes of pulse and coloring and the other observations he has made, he will proceed to set the patient in the most comfortable position possible. Then he will ask the patient to cough and will use this moment of distraction to insert the needle swiftly. The depth of insertion and the type of needle to be used are as punctiliously prescribed as are the length of time during which the needle has to remain *in situ,* and other relevant particulars. Some diseases require that the needle be left in the body for five minutes, others require a quarter of an hour, and others still longer.

Whether a puncture is to reduce a visceral plethora or whether it is to supplement a deficiency depends on the condition of the diseased organ. The list below gives instructions for the "correct" diagnosis of plethora and deficiency.

The Syndromes of Plethora (Excess) in the Internal Organs

Liver: Reddened eyes; dizziness; pains in the armpits; impaired hearing; disposition toward irritability; feeling of discontent.

Heart: Dry palate; flatulated diaphragm; pains in the back; tendency toward paroxysms of laughter (laughing fits).

Lungs: Respiratory difficulties; pains in the chest; gases in the upper parts of the body.

Kidneys: Sensation of heaviness throughout entire body; bloated abdomen; outbursts of perspiration after the consumption of food; aversion to speaking.

Stomach: Flatulent stomach and belly; constipation; immovability of the legs; quarrelsome moods.

Thy Syndromes of Deficiency in the Internal Organs

Liver: Brittleness of finger and toe nails; articular pains (pains in the joints); impaired vision; emotional insecurity and uneasiness.

Heart: Sciatic and lumbar pains; tightness in the root of the tongue; facial pallor; mental depression.

Lungs: Expectoration of blood; shortness of breath; emaciation.

Kidneys: Pains in the loins; swollen legs; fatigue; indecisiveness.

Stomach: Nausea; diarrhea; gastric cramps.

THE NEEDLES USED FOR ACUPUNCTURE

The classical school of acupuncture distinguishes nine types of needle. Their various shapes are said to have been invented by Emperor Huang-ti. The earliest needles were made of flint; later they were made of iron, gold, silver, copper, and other metals. Today, steel needles are used predominantly.

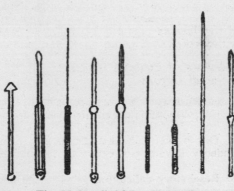

Fig. 55. Needles for acupuncture.

The nine classical shapes are:

1. The *Ch'an* needle, called arrow-headed because of the shape of its head. It is 1 *ts'un*, 6 *fen* long. Its upper point being ½ *ts'un* wide. It is employed mainly for skin diseases or fever-heat in the head, and is preferred for shallow punctures.

2. The *Yuan* needle is also 1 *ts'un*, 6 *fen* long. Its point is blunt and egg-shaped. It is most serviceable for "draining stagnant *pneuma* from amidst the flesh."

3. The *Shih* needle is 3 *ts'un*, 5 *fen* long. Its point resembles a millet seed. Its puncture forces stale *pneuma* to escape from the blood, thus providing room for healthy *pneuma*, and is recommended as a tonic. It should not be inserted very deeply.

4. The *Feng* needle is 1 *ts'un*, 6 *fen* long and has a three-cornered blade. Its use can diminish heat in the body, improve the circulation, and dilate the arteries. Among other diseases, it is applied in cases of leprosy.

5. The *Pi* needle is 4 *ts'un* long and 1½ *ts'un* wide. Its point resembles that of a short dagger. It is used particularly for draining pus from abscesses (hence actually an early surgical instrument).

6. The *Yüan-Li* needle is 1 *ts'un*, 6 *fen* long. Its point is round and slender. It is applied to replenish "vascular emptiness," to cure paralysis, rheumatism, and stagnation in the arteries.

7. The *Hao* needle is 3 *ts'un*, 6 *fen* long, and its point is as fine as hair. It helps to remove stale *pneuma* and cures light cases of paresthesia (abnormal spontaneous tingling, pricking, or numbness in various parts of the body). It may be allowed to penetrate deeply into the bone structure.

8. The *Chang* needle is also called the "long" needle, because of its length of 7 *ts'un*. It is designed for very deep punctures and is to be employed for curing tumors, including cancer.

9. The *Huo* needle (fire needle), 4 *ts'un* long, is used to alleviate congestions and swellings, and to cure poisonings.

THE MERIDIANS AND THE APPLICATION

OF THE PUNCTURES

The following pages and illustrations offer a deeper insight into the individual meridians and the actual application of acupuncture. The chart on pages 128–29, executed by H'sü Ch'ang, a famous old master of acupuncture, demonstrates the front part of the human body with the meridians visible on that side. The roman numerals in the listing below correspond to the numerals designating the meridians on the chart. The starting point of every meridian is marked *a* on the chart, and the end is marked *b*, so that the course of the meridian can be traced, for instance, from Ia to Ib. In cases where the beginning or end is not shown on the chart, the *a* or *b* is omitted.

The six Yin meridians:

I The *T'ai Yin* meridian of the hand (lung meridian) begins in the vicinity of the second rib and extends to the thumb (chart: Ia–Ib).

II The *Chüeh Yin* meridian of the hand (circulation meridian) begins just below the lung meridian, but slightly more toward the middle of the body, and runs to the terminal joint of the middle finger (chart: IIa–IIb).

III The *Shao Yin* meridian of the hand (heart meridian) begins above the armpit and reaches to the terminal joint of the little finger (chart: IIIa–IIIb).

IV The *Shao Lin* meridian of the foot (kidney meridian) begins in the middle of the sole and extends to the side of the breastbone, ending at a point between the first and second rib (figure 57, chart: IVa–IVb).

V The *Chüeh Yin* meridian of the foot (liver meridian) begins above the nailbed of the big toe and reaches upward to about two to three fingers below the mammilla (chart: Va–Vb).

VI The *T'ai Yin* meridian of the foot (spleen meridian) begins at the nailbed of the big toe and runs up to the area below the armpit (chart: VIa–VIb).

The six Yang meridians:

VII The *T'ai Yang* meridian of the hand (small-intestine meridian) begins at the nailbed of the little finger and extends to the opening of the external auditory canal (chart: VII–VII—a short stretch of it visible below the ears).

VIII The *Yang Ming* meridian of the hand (large-intestine meridian) begins above the nailbed of the index finger and runs up into the naso-labial fold (the muscular band between nose and upper lip) (figure 58, chart: VIII–VIIIb —becomes visible on forearms).

IX The *Shao Yang* meridian of the hand (three-warmers

meridian) begins above the nailbed of the ring finger and reaches up to the vicinity of the eyebrows (chart: IX–IXb —visible in area above ears).

X The *T'ai Yang* meridian of the foot (bladder meridian) begins at the flare of the nostrils, and extends over the top of the head and then all the way down to the bottom joint of the little toe (figure 59, chart: Xa–X—visible on face only).

XI The *Yang Ming* meridian of the foot (stomach meridian) begins at the side of the head, above the auricle, and extends down to above the nailbed of the second toe (chart: XIa–XI—disappears on thighs).

XII The *Shao Yang* meridian of the foot (gall-bladder meridian) reaches from the middle of the head down to the bottom joint of the little toe (chart: XIIa–XII, XII–XII— visible at temples, and again from shoulders to loins).

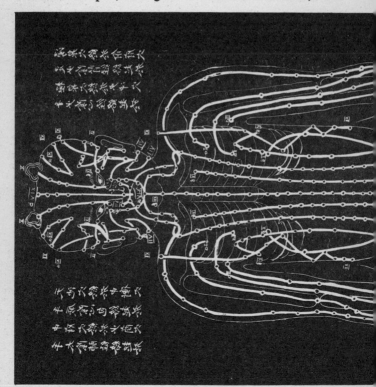

Two additional meridians:

XIII The *Jen*-vessel meridian begins at the pubis and reaches up to the middle of the upper lip (chart: XIIIa–XIIIb).

XIV The *Tu* meridian begins at the coccyx and extends up to the vertex of the head (chart: XIV–XIVb—visible on face).

Two examples may suffice to demonstrate which individual points are punctured for different maladies. The numbers listed refer to those which appear on the relevant illustration.

Hand-T'ai Yin—*Lung Meridian (figure 56)*

1. *Chung Fu:* Swollen joints; backaches; fever; pulmonary ailments; itching of skin.

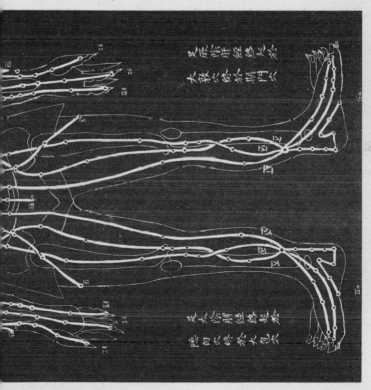

2. *Yün Men:* Excessive heat in joints; bronchitis; asthma; backaches.

3. *T'ien Fu:* Bleeding of the nose; pareses; mental depression; fever delirium; eye illnesses.

4. *Chia P'o:* Heart pains; short-windedness; vomiting.

5. *Ch'ih Tse:* Mental depression; crying fits; excessive urination (diuresis); coughing; swollen joints; asthma; lumbago (in child patients: infantile eclampsia, i.e., coma and convulsions).

6. *K'ung Tsui:* Incapability of stretching arm above the head; vomiting of blood; sore throat; headaches.

7. *Lieh Chüeh:* Weakness in arms; bloody diarrhea; pains in the genitals; swollen joints; pneumonia; spasms.

8. *Ching Ch'ü:* Heat in the palms of the hands; vomiting; fever; difficulty in emitting perspiration.

9. *T'ai Yüan:* Nausea; anxiety; insomnia; eye inflammations; respiratory disturbances; lung afflictions.

10. *Yü Chi:* Susceptibility to catarrhs; coated tongue; headaches; sore throat; restlessness.

11. *Shao Shang:* Chronic coughs; aching fingers; anxiety; hot palms.

Hand-Yang Ming—Large-Intestine Meridian (figure 58)

1. *Shang Yang:* Aching joints; coughs; fever without perspiration; toothache; hearing difficulties; eye weakness; sensitiveness to cold weather.

2. *Erh Chien:* Sore throat; backaches; cold in the nose; nose bleeding; neuralgia.

3. *San Chien:* Toothache; dry mouth; chapped lips.

4. *Ho Ku:* Incessant nose-bleeding; headache; high fever without perspiration; bloated face; speech disorders; (pregnant women must not receive stimulating puncture treatment).

5. *Yang Ch'i:* Irregular heartbeats; respiratory difficulties; fever; coughing; vomiting; eye afflictions.

6. *Pien Li:* Toothache; nose-bleeding; disorders in digestive and urinary tracts.

7. *Wen Liu:* Fever; headache; confused speech; swollen joints; sore throat; sensation of being persecuted by ghosts.

8. *Hsia Lien:* Bleeding of the bowels; rheumatism; facial pallor; bellyaches like the stab of knives; inflammation of the mammary gland; asthmatic breathing.

9. *Shang Lien:* Constricted urination; thoracic pains; neuralgia.

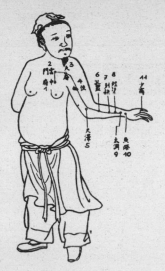

Fig. 56. Lung meridian.

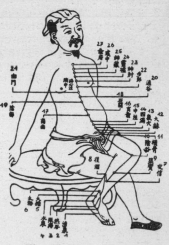

Fig. 57. Kidney meridian.

Fig. 58. Large-intestine meridian.

Fig. 59. Urinary-bladder meridian.

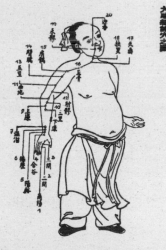

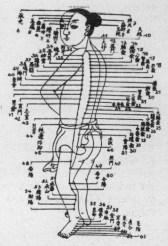

10. *San Li:* Toothache; pareses in arms and shoulders; feet and arms failing to function; heavy diarrhea; swollen glands.
11. *Ch'ü Ch'ih:* Pains in elbows; impediments of speech; fever; eczema; itching of skin; menstrual disorders.
12. *Chou Chia:* Fever; incapability of lifting arms.
13. *Wu Li:* Blood-coughing; immovability of limbs.
14. *Pei Nao:* Glandular swellings; fever; stiff shoulders and arms (for the above complaints, this point responds more favorably to moxibustion than to acupuncture).
15. *Chien Yü:* Enervated muscles; failing of arms and legs; heat in limbs.
16. *Chü Ku:* Blood-coughing; pains when stretching the arms.
17. *T'ien Ting:* Sore throat; dyspepsia.
18. *Fu Tu:* Coughing; excessive mucus in air ducts.
19. *Ho Chiao:* Lockjaw; adenoids; nose-bleeding; loss of the sense of smell.
20. *Ying Hsiang:* Swollen lips; short-windedness; stuffed nose; loss of sense of smell.

LISTING OF VARIOUS PUNCTURE POSSIBILITIES

Illness:	Meridians and Puncture Points to Be Treated:
Aching eyes:	large intestine: 5, 2
Eyes watering in the wind:	bladder: 2; large intestine: 4
Dulled eyesight:	bladder: 1, 2, 18, 23; large intestine: 4; lungs: 10
Swollen lips:	large intestine: 20
Coated tongue:	lungs: 10
Toothache:	large intestine: 1
Loss of hair:	large intestine: 8
Dry larynx, hoarseness:	lungs: 9, 10
Asthma:	lungs: 5
Blood-coughing:	large intestine: 13, 16; lungs: 1, 9
Arms ache and cannot be lifted:	large intestine: 3, 4, 10, 11, 15; lungs: 5, 9
Pains in elbows and arms:	large intestine: 10, 11, 15
Pains in palms and fingers:	lungs: 11
Hot palms:	kidney: 7, 8, 9
Mammillary ulcer:	large intestine: 8, 10; lungs: 10
Belly distended and aching:	lungs: 1; kidney: 1

Bellyaches:	kidney: 10, 8; bladder, 17, 20
Bowel gases:	large intestine: 10
Diarrhea with blood discharge:	lungs: 7; large intestine: 8
Backaches:	large intestine: 8, 10; bladder: 55, 59
Pains in lumbar area:	bladder: 49; kidney: 8
Pains in spinal column:	bladder: 27, 28, 49; kidney: 1
Weakness in legs:	bladder: 49, 52
Ice-cold feet:	bladder: 23
Skin-itching:	lungs: 1; large intestine: 11
Heat in the body:	large intestine: 11, 18; kidney: 8
Excessive perspiration:	first reducing in large intestine: 4 then stimulating in kidney: 8
Causeless bursts of perspiration:	large intestine: 11; lungs: 7, 11
Incapability of emitting perspiration:	lungs: 8, 10; large intestine: 2
Retention of perspiration:	first stimulating in large intestine: 4
Pustules over the entire body:	large intestine: 3, 4

CORRECT TIMING FOR THE APPLICATION

OF ACUPUNCTURE

At the risk of being accused of making naïve comparisons, the authors would like to point out that there are places in the West (for instance, Innsbruck in Austria), where surgical operations are postponed during certain atmospheric conditions, such as the foehn, which we have already mentioned. For the Chinese physician, it is an obvious principle that the needle may be applied only during certain time periods. Here are some of the concepts underlying that theory:

On a warm day full of clear sunshine, man's blood flows easily; his saliva protects his breath and keeps it light and swift; blood and breath circulate unobstructedly.

On cold days when the sun is clouded over, man's blood tends to condense and flow thickly through the blood vessels; his breath is deprived of its protection and keeps ebbing away. (According to the results of modern bioclimatic research, cases of coronary occlusion increase considerably during such weather.)

When the moon is waxing, man's blood and breath begin to circulate freely; his life essences protect his breath, so that it becomes mobile and active.

During the time of a full moon, man's blood and breath are copious; his muscles and flesh are firm.

When the moon is waning, man's muscles and flesh wane likewise and his arteries and veins are drained; his breath, no longer protected, becomes volatile and deserts the body.

The recognition of such facts makes it mandatory that one adjust one's treatment to time and weather conditions. In warm weather, acupuncture may be applied without hesitation; but when day or night are chilly, one should abstain from using it. Or, when a reducing puncture is applied during the period when sun and moon are waxing, it will weaken the patient's blood and breath; and when a stimulating puncture is performed at a full moon, then blood and breath will flow copiously and cause the blood in the veins to become congested.

The most favorable hours for stimulating and reducing punctures are as follows:

Lung meridian:
Stimulating	5–7 A.M.	point 9 of lung meridian
		(figure 56)
Reducing	3–5 A.M.	point 5 of lung meridian

Large-Intestine Meridian:
Stimulating	7–9 A.M.	point 11 of large-intestine meridian
		(figure 58)
Reducing	5–7 A.M.	point 2 of large-intestine meridian

Bladder Meridian:
Stimulating	5–7 P.M.	point 62 of bladder meridian
		(figure 59)
Reducing	3–5 P.M.	point 60 of bladder meridian

Kidney Meridian:
Stimulating	7–9 P.M.	point 8 of kidney meridian
		(figure 57)
Reducing	5–7 P.M.	point 1 of kidney meridian

To perform acupuncture during the period of the new moon means to induce confusion in the orderly flux of nature. *Yin* and *Yang* will be forced into combat, thus preventing a true diagnosis. The body's external channels will be depleted, causing internal plethora.

Undoubtedly, it was the practice of long and thorough observation of patients that led Chinese physicians to connect atmospheric changes with the causes and courses of diseases.

But since satisfactory and tangible explanations for man's sensitivity to weather were lacking, exalted concepts had to be introduced, or adapted, accordingly.

Even today, research in bioclimatology and the connection between medicine and the weather is still in its infancy. But who knows what fascinating revelations may be slumbering within these scientific fields, waiting to be detected for the entire realm of medical therapy?

ACUPUNCTURE WHEN FEVER IS PRESENT

If the fever begins by causing pains in thorax and pleura, and if hands and feet have become fidgety, then Foot-*Shao Yang* has to be reduced, and Foot-*T'ai Yin* stimulated.

But if the fever begins with pains in the hands and arms, then Hand-*Yang Ming* and Hand-*T'ai Yin* must be pricked until perspiration appears.

If the fever starts in the head, acupuncture has to be applied to the neck-point of the *T'ai Yang* meridian until perspiration appears.

If the fever emanates from thighs and shinbones, the Foot-*Yang Ming* must be pricked until perspiration appears.

Should the fever start with a sensation of heaviness throughout the body, with aching bones and hearing difficulties, Foot-*Shao Yin* has to be punctured. If the illness is severe, a great number of pricks must be made.

If bad vision and plethora in the chest and ribs accompany the beginning of fever, punctures have to be performed on Foot-*Shao Yin* as well as on Foot-*Shao Yang*.

Moxibustion

To bring *Yin* and *Yang* into proper balance is also the purpose of moxibustion—cauterization with moxa. While acupuncture is employed especially for diseases caused by an excess of *Yang*, the moxa method seeks to restrain an excess of *Yin*.

The most significant difference between the two remedies is that moxibustion is based on the therapeutic effect of heat, while acupuncture is a "cold" treatment. But many acupuncture points are said to respond to the moxibustion treatment also. However, the layman is urged to proceed very cautiously, since there are certain points that are absolutely taboo for moxa cautery, for instance, large-intestine point 2,

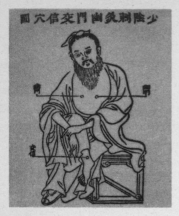

Fig. 60. Upper points: *Yü Men*, see fig. 57, point 21; lower point: *Chiao hsin*, see fig. 57, point 7.

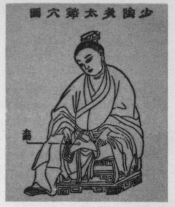

Fig. 61. Point *T'ai ch'i*, see fig. 57, point 6.

Fig. 62. Point *Ko Kuan*, kidney meridian at the back.

Fig. 63. Points for moxibustion in treating abscesses in the neck.

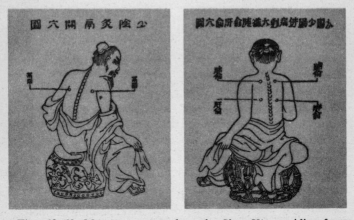

Figs. 60–62. Moxa treatment along the *Shao Yin* meridian for a disease of *Shao Yin* with the symptoms of cold hands and feet.

bladder points 1 and 49, and a considerable number of others.

To eliminate the danger of moxibustion at an unauthorized point, the Chinese doctor relies on drawings which mark clearly and unmistakably all points unfit for it.

The process of moxibustion as such presents no difficulty at all. The pulverized *Artemisia vulgaris* (wormwood) is kneaded into small cone-shaped lumps, which are set directly onto the point to be treated, ignited, and left to burn down to the very skin. It is customary to apply several cones simultaneously and to arrange them in a particular pattern.

Chinese medical textbooks warn against treating intoxicated persons with this cauterant. Where a pregnant woman is concerned, the physician should proceed with the utmost caution, since cauterization within certain segments of the body may damage the embryo. Here, as indeed in all other cases, only the skilled professional should be entrusted with the treatment. Administered judiciously to the correct points, moxibustion can bring considerable relief to a woman during delivery, so the moxa specialists claim. One of the effective points for moxibustion on pregnant women is the big toe. This point and a neighboring point between the big and second toes are equally suitable for the treatment of colics and heart pangs.

Pains below the ankle can be dispelled by cautery of point 57 of the bladder meridian (figure 59) and on point 3 of the kidney meridian (figure 57). An effective cure for putrid sores in the corner of the mouth is cautery on point 4 of the large-intestine meridian (figure 58). For boils on the hands, point 11 of the large-intestine meridian should be cauterized. If boils erupt over the entire body, moxibustion on points 3, 10 and 11 of the large-intestine meridian will make them heal. Children from 2 to 3 years old who suffer from reddened eyes and eyelids (catarrhal ophthalmia, a mild conjunctivitis) may be cured by moxibustion on the hand, in the space between the middle and index fingers.

Persons rescued from drowning should be stripped of their clothing immediately, and then moxibustion should be administered to the navel.

What is Western medicine's attitude toward the therapeutic use of cautery? Each burn, however tiny it may be, instigates a local irritation which may in its most extreme case lead to blood poisoning. For the sudden heat destroys the albumin; and the products of its decomposition are poisonous, so highly poisonous that extensive burns may be fatal. But as with every injury or extreme stress on the body, defensive enzymes become active; tissue serum is exuded; white blood corpuscles—the body's health guards—rush to the danger spot and literally devour the poisonous debris. In the course of the battle, the white corpuscles usually perish themselves and are carried off as refuse—suppuration—in some form or other.

The Western healing method most closely resembling moxibustion is perhaps dry cupping. In wet cupping—an age-old "suction treatment"—the skin is scratched with a knife or a scarificator (an instrument containing several small lancets); then a cupping glass is turned over and pressed on the spot, and blood and tissue serum are drawn to the surface and removed. In dry cupping, which is preferred to this day as a draining treatment on patients who are over-sensitive to modern diuretics, the glass is turned onto the unbroken surface and the skin is sucked until a distinct blister has formed.

In moxibustion and in acupuncture, as in neurotherapy, it is undoubtedly of significance to be exact in choosing the spot to which the treatment is applied, since it determines the nerve-area in which the defensive actions concentrate. Unfortunately, no thorough treatises exist as yet on the effects of moxibustion, which may be superior to acupuncture in certain cases, since it stimulates a more extensive area.

Massage

The aforementioned Head's zones also constitute the chief areas for massage of the connective tissue. Startling results are again being achieved with this old traditional therapy; and it seems odd indeed that for a long time it was left to barber-surgeons and unskilled persons to keep this tradition alive.

In China, massages have been appreciated as therapeutic treatment since ancient times. One may safely assume that the knowledge of the zones of "referred pain" was even then put to good use. During the T'ang Dynasty, a period of high achievement in the field of medicine, the art of massage was taught in specially founded institutes.

The simpler hand movements of massage are known to almost every Chinese. Thus it is taken for granted that a devoted daughter-in-law will refresh her revered mother-in-law with a quick massage when the latter is low and fatigued.

Boys perform the same service for their fathers and grandfathers. From China the art of massaging spread into other eastern countries and finally into Japan, where it was developed and refined still further.

Exercises for Prolonging Life

Correct breathing is the basis of all exercises recommended in China for longevity, as well as for the cure of several diseases. As early as the fourth century B.C., the philosopher Chuang-tzu (fl. c. 400–370) promulgated that men of great wisdom fetch their breath from deep inside and below, while ordinary men breathe with the larynx alone. In other words, men were even then aware of the great value of deep respiration.

The principal purpose of Chinese gymnastic exercises, as is the purpose of the Indian Yoga practices, is to attain proper circulation of the blood which, in turn, will ensure emotional balance and stability. This stability is to lend the body resistance against illnesses and consequently grant a longer life. Correct breathing is also mentioned very early as a means of cleansing the blood and body of their debris. Congestions may be removed and stiff joints limbered by adhering to the pertinent exercise instructions.

Contrary to many Yoga practices, Chinese exercises are quite simple throughout and demand neither particular exertion nor extraordinary and violent bodily contortions. Still, perseverance and strong will-power are indispensable if one wants to attain the final goal. All details are prescribed minutely, from the body posture to the exact position and motion of the fingers, and they have to be followed methodically. Such exercises can be performed accurately only under the supervision of an instructor, who watches each movement carefully. Very similar practices are to be found in Japan, especially in Zen Buddhism.

Under no circumstances must therapeutic or life-prolonging gymnastics lead to tenseness, let alone exhaustion. On the contrary, the aim is to relax physiological and psychological tension and to strengthen the life-impulses.

To assure adequate concentration, care must be taken that the exercising person is not distracted by anything. The most propitious hours are therefore the early morning hours, before the day awakes with its distracting clamor. All exercises must be performed on an empty stomach. For each month, certain drills are prescribed, which have to be repeated several times. During the repetitions, it is most important that the prescribed pauses between the drills are obeyed closely also, in order to keep a balanced body rhythm.

Here are some examples of the exercises:

Exercise for the third month: To be practiced daily during the hours from 1 to 3 A.M. (figure 64).

While sitting with crossed legs and with the back held absolutely straight, the exerciser bends one arm and stretches the other, as though he is bending a very stiff bow. This movement is to be repeated seven to eight times with each arm.

The exercise is designed to refresh depleted kidneys and stomach, and to alleviate stiffness in neck and shoulders. It is recommended for all people who have difficulty in bending down. The blood circulation is stimulated, which diminishes susceptibility to colds. Congestions are dissolved. People with aural defects will regain their hearing.

Exercise for the fifth month: To be practiced daily during the hours from 3 to 5 A.M. (figure 66).

One stands erect, legs slightly apart, and bends the upper body backward very slowly as far as possible. Now, with palms turned outward, both arms are raised above the head simultaneously and with force, and then lowered to the sides of the body. To be repeated five to six times.

This is said to be a very effective drill for curing uncontrollable thirst, as well as pains in heart, hips, and neck. It soothes hoarseness and coughs, and influences the emotional disposition equally well. Mental depression, as well as impaired memory and nervous jumpiness, will be mitigated.

Exercise for the sixth month: To be performed daily between 1 and 3 A.M. (figure 67).

In a kneeling position, put both hands flat on the floor, keeping the back erect. One leg at a time is now stretched out in front to its full length and then pulled back energetically. To be repeated three to five times with each leg.

This exercise will dispel the effects of dampness and wind on the spleen, the hips, the knees, and the sacroiliac. It is highly recommended for rheumatism, asthma, and heaviness in the limbs. Beyond that, it exerts a favorable influence on the emotions.

Exercise for the seventh month: To be performed daily between 1 and 3 A.M. (figure 68).

Sit with legs crossed and back perfectly straight; the head

should be turned sharply to the right and to the left while both fists simultaneously drum on the back. To be performed five to six times to either side.

If executed properly, this drill will disperse congestions in the thorax and remove coughs. It is recommended for sciatica as well as for pains in chest, back, ribs, in the coccyx, the knees, and the ankles.

Exercise for the tenth month: To be practiced daily between 1 and 3 A.M. (figure 69).

Sit erect with legs crossed; the neck has to be held quite stiff and must be turned as far as possible first to one side,

Fig. 64. Exercise for the third month. Fig. 65. Concentration exercise for the fourth month. Fig. 66. Exercise for the fifth month.

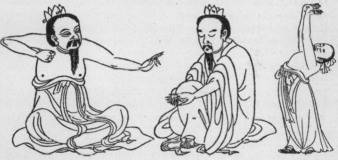

Fig. 67. Exercise for the sixth month. Fig. 68. Exercise for the seventh month. Fig. 69. Exercise for the tenth month.

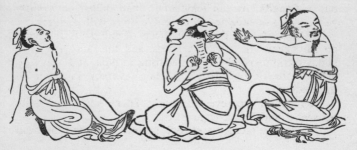

then to the other. At the same time, the arms are held out in front of the body and are moved in the opposite direction from that of the head. To be repeated three to five times.

This is an effective exercise for congestions in chest and ribs, for aches in head and sacroiliac, for stiffness when bending down, for deafness, and for hoarseness. Also lessens proneness to vomiting and diarrhea.

Concentration exercise for the fourth month: To be performed daily between 3 and 5 A.M. (figure 65).

Sit down, close your eyes, and inhale deeply. Then, while holding your breath, embrace one knee with both hands, palms turned outward and fingers interlaced, and pull up the knee. Then repeat this with the other knee. Five to seven times with each leg.

This exercise serves to overcome emotional disquiet and restlessness and forces one to concentrate. In addition, it relieves pains in arms, armpits, and wrists. It can also expel heat from the palms.

The perceptions inherent in Indian and Chinese physical and respiratory exercises are quite consonant with the latest results of Western research. That Western man may yet have to learn an immense amount in this respect is demonstrated rather clearly in a work by J. Schmitt, *Atemheilkunst* (*The Art of Therapeutic Breathing*), in which the matter devotes one richly illustrated chapter to Yoga exercises.

Orthopedic Treatment Methods

When until recently in the Western world children were strapped into all sorts of stretching devices, our orthopedic treatment methods were in no way different from those prescribed by Chinese physicians. Figures 70 and 71 convey how back supports are attached to a patient. One (seen in figure 70) is made of two pine boards, approximately 3 *ts'un* wide and 2 *ts'un* long, which extend about 1 *ts'un* over the shoulderblades, measured from the waist. The outer board is even and flat on the outside, while the inner board is concave on the side that touches the back. Along each side of the outer board, five holes are drilled, and two top ones fairly close together, the other three at an equal, longer distance from each other. Through these holes, ribbons are laced with which the contraption is tied to its wearer. Before strapping it on, the patient's body has to be protected with thick layers of cotton.

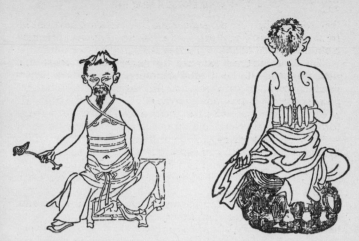

Figs. 70 and 71. Spinal supports, front and back views.

Fig. 72. Splint for a fracture in the forearm.

Fig. 73. Stretching device for affections of the spinal column.

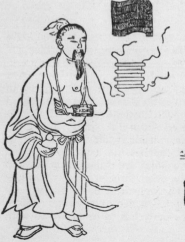

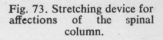

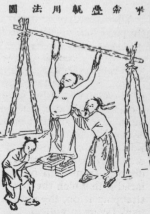

The modern traction treatment with the jury mast (an upright bar with a sling in which the chin rests) that is employed for strengthening and straightening the spinal column, as well as other extension equipment, was anticipated by a Chinese apparatus for the same purpose. The Chinese device (see figure 73) consists of a racklike structure made of sturdy logs and two strong rope slings suspended from its crossbar. Two piles of three bricks each are placed a few inches apart under the crossbar. The patient steps on these bricks and grabs the rope slings with both hands. Then, while one assistant supports the patient's back, another carefully pulls one brick after another from underneath the patient's feet. With each removal of a brick, the patient is forced to stretch his back a bit more. How many bricks are finally removed depends on the severity of the patient's condition.

The ingenuity and appropriateness of the splint for a forearm fracture—which is clearly depicted in the drawings of figure 72, full-view and close-up—are staggering. Since the plaster cast was not known at that time (and, in any case, usually makes X-ray equipment necessary), this Chinese method of splinting must be regarded as the ideal solution. Only the position of the sling is inappropriate. The band should, of course, be slung around the splint, rather than pull on the hand as shown; but this could very likely be an error on the part of the illustrator.

Talismans

Chinese medical therapy avails itself not only of medications, of color and other correspondences, and of the treatment possibilities decreed by the natural rhythm of the seasons. The Chinese doctor also draws upon the magical powers of talismans, even to this day.

These talismans are for the most part ideographs similar to the characters of common Chinese writing and are painted in black on a background of yellow or red paper. For the talisman characters, however, a special form of brush-stroke writing exists.

Each disease has its own particular exorcising charm, which is expressed in the written symbol. One of them is shown in figure 74; this talisman was employed against the epidemic of 1907.

The talismans are either tied to the patient's bed, or they are burnt and the ashes swallowed by the patient.

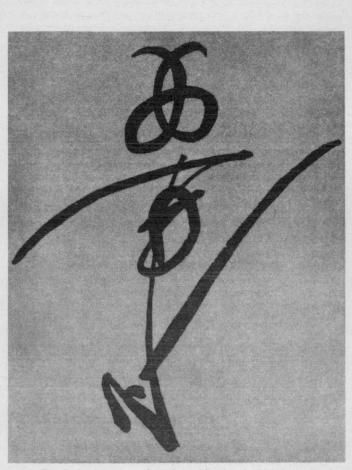

Fig. 74. Talisman against the epidemic of 1907. It says,
"Protect us, ye five gods of the dome!"

It is interesting to note in this respect that in Taoistic and Buddhist temples one does not pray to have an illness cured, but begs to be presented with the correct remedy for it. To this end, small rolls containing prescriptions are tossed together and are then picked by the supplicants, as in a lottery.

VII

AGING AND DYING

The Death of Mr. Wu

Mr. Wu's bereaved family were kneeling in front of the table on which was placed the soul-chest of the clan. The bonzes had opened the chest wide, so that the dead man's soul could find its way back into it. Mr. Wu's three sons, with tears in their voices, assured the assembled family how gladly they would have died in their father's stead, had they been able to save his life by doing so.

Clad in their white mourning robes, the relatives stood quietly and gazed admiringly at the splendid coffin, which was made of carefully selected wood and which father Wu to his utmost joy had been given as a present when he was still very much alive. His shroud, also, had been selected and measured to his body years ago by his loving sons.

Now he lay quiet and peaceful, surrounded by houses, valets and chambermaids, horses, sedan chairs, and sacrificial food dishes—all of it neatly cut out of paper and ready to accompany him on his journey to the beyond, in order that he should not lack anything there.

Some time ago, the *Fen Shui* Master had chosen the appropriate spot for the grave, with the help of his geomantic compass. And now that the blessed day had arrived—also prophesied by the geomancer—the beloved departed man could be carried to his last place of rest in festive procession, accompanied by the ringing sounds of gongs and music.

"The calling back of the soul is the manner in which love is demonstrated. It is the expression of the voice of prayer," says the ancient *Li Chi*.

As ancient is the tradition of placing objects and food dishes in the coffin with the dead. "To fill the mouth, rice and mussels must be laid inside," states again the *Li Chi*. The custom of enclosing the dead person's favorite objects in his coffin has been maintained to this day. The artist Chi P'ai Shih, who died in 1958 at the age of more than ninety years, begged his family to bury him with his brushes beside him.

147

Signs of Impending Death

When the bones in a man's body have become brittle and are decomposing, and when the flesh sags, then the chest fills itself with gases and breathing becomes troubled. When the person is unable to urinate in this condition and when he cannot dislodge the gases within him, death will overtake him six months hence.

When the bones are brittle, when the flesh sags, when the chest is filled with gases, when breathing becomes difficult and the person tries in vain to urinate, then internal pains will be created. When such pains then advance up into the shoulders and into the nape of the neck, death will occur one month later. But if beyond that the heart pulse is deficient, death will strike the very same day.

When the bones in the body have become brittle and the flesh sags, when the chest is filled with gases, when breathing has become difficult and urinating impossible, when pains have developed within and have advanced into the shoulders and the nape of the neck, then fever-heat may arise within the body. When beyond that the flesh withers away at the elbows and behind the knees and the pulse of the spleen is debilitated, then death will occur in ten months.

When the bones have become brittle and the flesh sags, when the marrow in the shoulder bones has disintegrated and the person's movements become more and more unco-ordinated, when the pulse of the kidney begins to deteriorate, then death will occur in a year. But if the kidney pulse is extremely devastated, then the patient will die on the very same day.

When the bones have become brittle and the flesh sags, when the chest is filled with gases, when pains appear in the abdomen and within the heart, when shoulders and neck are feverish and the flesh at the elbows and behind the knees has decomposed, then the eyes will sink in. When beyond that the pulse of the liver becomes hard, then the eyes will no longer recognize anybody and death will strike at once.

The Meridians and Death

If death is induced by *T'ai Yang*, then the eye stares fix-edly and is turned upward. Spasms will occur, and the patient's complexion is white. Perspiration will erupt suddenly, and when all perspiration has left the body, death occurs.

When death is induced by *Shao Yang,* then the ear goes deaf, all the joints become limp, and the eye can no longer perceive its surroundings, because all vital connections have been disrupted. The complexion turns green abruptly, then white, and after one and one half days death will occur. (*Shao Yang* also governs the bones, hence the failure of the joints.)

When death is induced by *Yang Ming,* then mouth and eyes may still be moved fairly easily, but the patient is tormented by fitful frights and speaks incoherently. His face turns sallow as the color of earth; upper and lower meridians are full and congested and function no more. Now death will strike.

When death is induced by *Shao Yin,* then the patient's complexion becomes black, his teeth become longish and putrid. The abdomen is distended and its orifices are blocked up. Upper and lower circulation ceases. Life is extinguished.

When death is induced by *T'ai Yin,* then the abdomen is distended and blocked up. The patient will gasp for breath, wheeze, and vomit. This will make his complexion turn red. When circulation ceases, his face will turn black. Skin and body-hair are desiccated, and the end is approaching.

When death is induced by *Chüeh Yin,* then the larynx is hot and dry. The heart is agitated. The tongue curls back. The patient dies.

Geomancy—The Art of Divining by Earthlines and Rays

The selection of a suitable spot for the grave before one dies is an ancient tradition. There are tomes of writings about the manner in which a burial place must be laid out in order to afford the most perfect compliance with the principles of *Yin* and *Yang,* and in order to receive the breath of the universe properly from all sides. Not only grave sites, but homes, as well as gardens, have been laid out according to these concepts since time immemorial.

The scope of *Fen Shui*—geomancy—presents a wide field of study all on its own. It comprises divination based on the extension of underground watercourses, the presence and location of mountains in the vicinity, and countless other geographic details. Last, but not least, the geomancer has to make certain that it will be impossible for evil demons to sneak up and into the home, the garden, the field, or the grave.

It is not the concern of this book to examine whether all research studies on the so-called earth rays are without exception charlatanry. Be it merely mentioned here, with the utmost caution, that there are areas on this planet that are totally exempt from certain diseases. Such zones have reportedly been discovered even within Europe. This statement is not to be read as favoring quacks and frauds. But it does seem indisputable that there are some genuine and successful dowsers, for industry and agriculture are constantly taking advantage of their water-divining powers.

Perhaps the system by which the Chinese geomancers operate is based on principles similar to those on which dowsing seems to work. Here, as there, however, their more excessive claims should be banished into the realm of fantasy and mass deception.

Allowing that the master geomancer merely used his life's experience coupled with common sense in appointing the proper spots for houses, fields, and graves, allowing that he only followed directions inherited from his ancestors and teachers, who simply advised him against constructing houses in swampy areas, it does not alter the fact that geomancers were held in the highest esteem, and there was hardly a Chinese alive who would not avail himself of their services and advice if he could at all afford them.

This may not be so far-fetched if we call to mind that throughout man's history, hygienic necessity has often been clad in the robes of religion—mostly, it goes without saying, to the benefit of the faithful believers (one has to remember only the rules against eating pork, or the practice of circumcision).

The obstinate adherence to geomantic rules on the part of the Chinese has sometimes proved a great obstacle to Western engineers. Wherever the latter intended to lay tracks for a railroad construction, some "unfavorable" spot was sure to lie on the route. And any altering of the landscape would have catastrophic consequences—according to the geomancers.

VIII

TORTURES AS

"PILLARS OF JUSTICE"

Wu Chiang Tu, the Thief

Wu Chiang Tu, well-known robber and bandit, had made a splendid catch. Last night, very late, there was that old man who came strolling down the path unsuspectingly, with his money bag filled to the brim. Clever Wu Chiang Tu, who had lain hidden behind the bushes, shot out like a dart, threw himself on the man, tore his purse from him, and escaped with the booty. But what he did not see was that the old fellow was so petrified with fright that his heart stood still and he collapsed and died on the spot.

Exhilarated with joy over his success, Wu Chiang Tu called together his friends and invited them to a sumptuous feast in a tavern. But his generosity had drawn attention to him; and when the old man's body was found the next day, our villain was arrested and at once subjected to torture in order to press a confession out of him.

The kneeling on iron chains was nothing new to Wu Chiang Tu, nor were the one hundred lashes with the whip that they let him have. But when they began to crush together his ankles, he finally broke down and confessed his evil deed.

During the successive periods of the Chou and the Han dynasties (1122 B.C.–A.D. 220), five degrees of punishment were known:

1. Branding the forehead with a hot iron: For petty infractions of the law of various kinds.
2. The nose cut off: For willfully damaging traveling coaches or garments; for theft.

3. The ears, hands, feet cut off; removal of the knee-caps:

For burglary; for damaging bridges or city gates.

4. Castration:

For abduction; adultery; robbery with murder; for high treason (as a penalty for high treason, the historian Sze Ma Chien was castrated around A.D. 100).

5. Death (mostly by strangling):

For murder and for high treason; also for drunkenness.

Castration, however, was not always used as a punishment. As in some other parts of the world, it was performed also in order to provide eunuchs for the Emperor's women's quarters.

History tells of a usurper of the beginning of the tenth century A.D. who reveled in extremely perverse brutalities. If the face of a person displeased him, the poor wretch was flung into prison and submitted to the most excruciating tortures. Either he had to stand over his hips in fetid water, crammed in so tightly with other unfortunates that he could not budge; or writhing bundles of poisonous snakes were thrown into his dungeon cell. The grandson and successor of this gentleman even surpassed him. He would release wild beasts to attack the prisoners, or he had them chased over a hill made of the sharpened blades of daggers.

It was around the same period that several new types of punishment appeared, for instance, a person convicted of high treason, the murder of a parent, or adultery was chopped to pieces. Other known methods were: suspending the criminal from his thumb, crushing together the ankles (reserved for men), squeezing together the fingers (for men and women), slapping the mouth until the teeth were loosened, twisting off the ear, making the criminal kneel on chains, and many other cruelties. These methods of torturing were practiced not only on the criminal himself, but also on his accomplices.

During the Ch'ing Dynasty (1644–1912), the five aforementioned degrees of punishment were altered as follows:

1. Beating with the bamboo rod:

5 degrees of intensity

2. Beating with clubs:

5 degrees of intensity

3. Exile:

5 degrees of time-period to be exiled

4. Exile for life: 3 degrees of distances
5. Death through strangling
    or beheading.

Frequently also the method of *Ling cho,* the "tantalizing death," was employed. As its name implies, this method consisted of having a possible death dangling before the convict constantly. By some abhorrent and ingenious device, the delinquent was liberated from his torment just at the moment when he wanted desperately to die—only to be submitted to more and worse tortures the next day.

IX

THE TORTURES OF FASHION

—COSMETICS

One sometimes reads with surprise of the immense amount of money spent by the women of the modern world on their make-up. In Old China it was little different. Perfume, powder, and cream make-up were beloved everywhere and used extensively, and the dictatorship of fashion often ruled more relentlessly than it does today. Even men took great pains to preserve their complexion.

The war god Kuan Yün, whom we met in the section headed Famous Doctors and Famous Works, even went so far as to have a special casing made to protect his beard.

After a meal, hot wet towels were applied to the face—and still are, as any frequenter of Chinese restaurants will attest to readily. These steamy compresses are supposed to prevent the early forming of wrinkles.

Red nail-polish was known in China a long time before it became fashionable in the West. The coloring agent used at that time was the juice of the *T'u ku* herb (literally: the herb that penetrates to the very bones). This juice made the nails a very deep, glowing red and had the advantage of adhering to the nails for a long time. Until very recently it was considered particularly dignified to have nails over an inch long. To prevent the breaking and chipping of such elegant claws, tiny protective shields of silver would be fastened over them.

It was almost incomprehensible for Western minds that the cruel fashion of crippling women's feet could have endured in China for so many centuries. Not merely the leisure class, but even peasant girls had their feet mutilated and therefore were compelled to perform their work on their knees most of the time; standing would have meant excruciating pain.

Many different stories are told about the origin of that freak of fashion. One version has it that Pao-Kuan, the fair and favorite mistress of the Emperor who ruled around A.D.

500, once danced over a carpet strewn with lilies, until the Emperor exclaimed rapturously: "Is it not as though the lilies were bursting forth from under every one of her steps?"

Since the graceful dancer had especially dainty little feet, all of the Emperor's concubines henceforth bandaged their feet, so that they might equal those of the dancer. From this version stems the name "the fashion of the golden lily," by which this practice is sometimes known.

One learns to appreciate the Chinese saying "each pair of bandaged feet means a bathful of tears," when one hears how the bandaging was done to the feet of the wretched children. When a girl was only four to five years old, the torture began. The bandage was wound around the foot so tightly that the child was just able to endure the pain. The big toe was left free, but all the other toes were folded under the sole. Each morning and evening, the bandages were pulled tighter, and the little girls had to patter back and forth several times in order to prevent gangrene from setting in. During subsequent years, the bandages were gradually pulled so tight that the fleshy parts of the feet were eventually pressed close to the heels.

Finally, the space between the heel and the ball of the foot would get so narrow that even a coin could be inserted only with force. Only when that was achieved were the feet considered fully perfected. Although Emperor K'ang Hsi (1654–1722) had issued an edict forbidding mothers to mutilate their daughters' feet, this bad practice remained widespread and was only finally abolished after the establishment of the Chinese Republic in 1912.

Rather ironically, the shoes into which those abused feet of women and girls were finally squeezed were often veritable works of art, with imaginative embroidery in gold or precious jewels.

But let us not forget that we have a Western counterpart to this, too. The wasp-waist, forced into thinness by tightly laced corsets, stays, and bodices, was the ideal image of a beautiful woman only about fifty or so years ago. The constriction of the waist caused all sorts of liver ailments; and if one were to read through the doctors' manuals of old, one would probably find any number of descriptions and illustrations of such a maltreated liver.

But the narrow waist is by no means a Western invention. It is historically documented that around the year 1100 B.C., Chinese ladies were already dying of starvation because a wasp-waistline was deemed by them more valuable than life itself.

X

TALES, DREAMS, AND

THEIR INTERPRETATIONS

THE DREAM OF PRINCE CHING

Prince Ching was suffering from dropsy and was confined to his bed. Ten days after the outbreak of his illness, the patient had a most disturbing dream. The following morning, he immediately sent for his court councillor, Yen Tze. The Prince feared that the dream contained a bad omen, perhaps even the beckoning of death. Yen Tze urged him to relate his dream.

"I dreamed," the Prince began, "that I was fighting with two suns that dominated the sky. But although I fought with all my strength, I could not defeat them. I am frightened, for this may be a sign that I shall have to die soon," the Prince sighed.

"I beg your pardon most humbly, Your Royal Highness, when I differ from your opinion. Your illness is a malady of the *Yin* nature. The two suns are the symbols of *Yang*. One *Yin* alone is not adequate to destroy two *Yang* substances. *Yang* will retain its potency. You will soon recover." Three days later, the Prince had regained his full health.

The renowned scholar Yen Tze, as is evident, had recognized instantly that the *Yin* disease of the Prince had already reached its crisis point, that *Yang* was already rising within the body of the patient and had begun to regain its vigor. A total cure was the logical prognosis.

To prophets and scholars, but also to magicians and charlatans of all types, the world of dreams has always been a singular and unique realm, whose boundaries defy exact definition. The unreasoned fear of the unconscious, or subconscious, may have contributed to the obstinate resistance that Sigmund Freud encountered among his colleagues. It is said that he was never permitted to address the illustrious society

156

of Viennese physicians; in fact, that he never even entered their chambers.

His *Interpretation of Dreams*, written for the medical profession, was read by "a wider circle of educated and curious-minded readers," as he himself stated in his preface to the second edition.* In other words, it was read by that circle of people that the reactionaries of all eras have always regarded with suspicion. It was only much later that the professional world realized that Freud's book was not a "dreambook" in the ordinary sense.

Freud himself writes in the opening chapter of his work:

"In the pages that follow I shall bring forward proof that there is a psychological technique which makes it possible to interpret dreams, and that, if that procedure is employed, every dream reveals itself at an assignable point in the mental activities of waking life. I shall further endeavor to elucidate the processes to which the strangeness and obscurity of dreams are due and deduce from those processes the nature of the psychical forces by whose concurrent or mutually opposing action dreams are generated. Having gone thus far, my description will break off, for it will have reached a point at which the problem of dreams merges into more comprehensive problems, the solution of which must be approached upon the basis of material of another kind."†

The interpretation of dreams on the basis of physical stimuli and normal mental processes is part of Freud's endeavor. We quote him again here:

"Incidentally, it would be a mistake to suppose that the theory of the supernatural origin of dreams is without its supporters in our own days. We may leave on one side pietistic and mystical writers, who, indeed, are perfectly justified in remaining in occupation of what is left of the once wide domain of the supernatural so long as that field is not conquered by scientific explanation. But apart from them, one comes across clear-headed men, without any extravagant ideas, who seek to support their religious faith in the existence and activity of superhuman spiritual forces precisely by the inexplicable nature of the phenomena of dreaming."‡

An endless amount of new material has been added to Freud's discoveries in the years since they were made. With such recent knowledge in mind, we cannot help but wonder when studying the ancient sages—who were often excellent

* *Interpretation of Dreams,* translated by James Strachey, © 1955 by Basic Books, Inc., Publishers, New York City.

† *Ibid.*

‡ *Ibid.*

psychologists without the background of the science of psychology as such—whether they did not know more about the problems of the human soul than they ever wanted to transmit to their disciples and posterity. But anyway, there are probably mysteries within the human domain that can only be conceived intuitively and can never be constrained into the pages of a book, but can at best, perhaps, hover between the lines.

Therefore, to the discerning mind, Chinese fables must likewise appear as more than sheer fairy tales, and it is for this reason that they are included in the pages of this book. To the psychoanalyst, moreover, folk myths and legends are ever welcome starting material to those attempting to interpret the nature of a people's emotional disposition.

There are two separate categories of myths living alongside each other in China: one group has a distinct Buddhist influence, the others are purely Chinese folktales. In the former, the concept of reincarnation naturally plays the predominant role. In the folktales, one recurrent theme is that of a dead girl who is resurrected from her grave, falls in love with a young man, and visits him nightly; and another very popular one is the fox theme: the nightly visitor is really a vixen, who, in the disguise of a beautiful maiden, ensnares the young man, lures him into her arms, and then gradually draws the blood out of him, as a vampire does.

The original source of the vixen myth, which is also widespread throughout Japan, has never been satisfactorily explained. In several other versions of it, the main characters are male foxes, disguised as kindly old gentlemen, who are endowed with the mesmeric powers of magi.

A tale of the Buddhist class from the *Liao Chai Chih I,* a collection of folktales by Pu Su Ling, concerns a scholar who after his death is brought before the Prince of the Underworld. In punishment for his misdeeds on earth, the scholar is sentenced to spend his new life in the form of a sheep. But just as the spirits of hell are preparing to pull the sheep's fleece over him, one of the demons happens to recall one good deed done by the delinquent. Instantly they try to pull away the sheepskin, but too late: parts of it have already grown together with the man's own skin. And so, even after his reincarnation as a human being, one small piece of sheepskin was forever to be visible on his shoulder.

Thus the little story, unassuming enough. But perhaps it harbors a deeper psychological insight? Could not the scrap of sheepskin be an old guilt-feeling which remains in the consciousness, or subconsciousness, of a person even after he is rehabilitated before the world? Do we not know only too well today of the existence of guilt complexes—often not even justified by an actual misdeed, but nonetheless weaving like threads in and out of a man's life until they become the cause of his neurosis?

There is also a tale of the fox myth type, from the *Liao Chai Chih I*. A young lad is visited every night by an enchantingly pretty girl. Although he senses that she is really a vixen, he is not able to escape her charm. His parents are despondent when they see him pine away more and more as the days go by. By fastening talismans to his bed, they hope to prevent the vixen-girl from returning, but all attempts are of no avail. Only when the father finally decides to sleep at the youth's side in his bed does the vixen declare that she will henceforth stay away: "It would be unbefitting to come to thee at night in the presence of thy father."

The young man recovers. But a short while thereafter, riots break out in the village, in the course of which our hero has to flee up into the mountains to hide himself. Suddenly, the beauty appears again and announces that she will now build him a house. No sooner said than done; after a few minutes, a splendid palace is standing before him, although entirely without windows and doors. The couple now spend an unforgettable night in love and rapture. When the young man awakens the next morning, the palace has disappeared, and so has the vixen. But where the palace has stood, there is now a ring lying on the ground, with four needles stuck in it.

It would not only be contrary to this book's professed intentions, but also absolutely against all the principles of Chinese folklore, were we not to leave it to each individual reader to interpret the tales according to his own insights.

The interpretation of dreams is an age-old science for the Chinese. Just as today's psychoanalyst lets his patients recount their dreams in order to draw his conclusions from them, so did the sages of ancient times. And it seems justified to assume that those conclusions were often akin to the sober diagnoses of our times.

The Dream-Principles of "Yin" and "Yang"

When *Yin* is predominant, then a person will dream of wading through great water-floods, whilst being weary with anguish and fears. When *Yang* is dominant, then a person will dream that he is being consumed by a raging fire. When both *Yin* and *Yang* are equally strong, dreams will occur of heavy battles and violence.

When the upper pulse is abundant, one dreams of flying. When the lower pulse is abundant, one dreams of falling into an abyss.

An excess of *Ch'i* in the liver will produce nightmares.

An excess of *Ch'i* in the heart will produce joyous dreams.

An excess of *Ch'i* in the lungs will produce dreams of anxiety and sorrow.

An excess of *Ch'i* in the spleen will produce oppressive dreams.

An excess of *Ch'i* in the kidneys will produce dreams of worms and wounds.

A deficiency of *Ch'i* in the liver will induce dreams of lying under a tree and being unable to rise, dreams of grass and sprouting wheat.

A deficiency of *Ch'i* in the heart will create dreams of being rescued from flames of fire, dreams of the sun and of success.

A deficiency of *Ch'i* in the lungs will produce dreams of fighting, of white objects and of beheadings.

A deficiency of *Ch'i* in the spleen will bring forth dreams of hunger and thirst and of the construction of houses and walls.

A deficiency of *Ch'i* in the kidneys will produce dreams of shipwrecks and drowning.

In conclusion, let us compare these dream-principles of *Yin* and *Yang* with the findings of Freud: "Any complete enumeration of the sources of dreams leads to a recognition of four kinds of sources; and these have also been used for the classification of dreams themselves. They are:

1. external (objective) sensory excitations;
2. internal (subjective) sensory excitations;
3. internal (organic) somatic stimuli;
4. purely psychical sources of stimulation."*

* *Ibid.*

XI

AN END AND A BEGINNING

From the wisdom and discoveries of the *Nei Ching* and Lao-tzu to Sigmund Freud and his rediscovery of the unconscious, a long bridge extends which, alas, has been used but rarely for the traffic and exchange of ideas. Yet, the bridge exists. But what has kept it aloft is probably all the individuals in East and West who, though unknown to one another, have been searching for the same thing: the meaning and purpose of life beyond daily needs and narrow domestic boundaries. And the conclusions that each has arrived at in his search appear different from the others' conclusions only on the surface.

How close the kinship is between Eastern and Western basic beliefs and emotional needs may be demonstrated by the life-work of the philosopher Mo Ti (also called Mo-tzu), who lived during the fifth century B.C. Mo Ti not only spoke liberally about God's love for men, but also urged his disciples and followers to promote universal love among the people themselves. As Mo Ti says, "if (only) all of man's society could be brought together in an all-embracing love . . . " And it should not surprise us to hear that Mo Ti's doctrines were as little obeyed in China as the demand "love thy neighbor as thyself" was obeyed by the "Western barbarians." But the demand is becoming more and more imperative for man of the atomic age, be he doctor, clergyman, or teacher with a direct influence on man's education, or be he simply a "neighbor."

By no means should we cast aside any help or advice that Chinese philosophy may be able to offer us. Certainly not all of it is superstition and demon cult. The realm of medicine especially could profit from a closer scrutiny of some of the ancient healing methods. Much beneficial truth may be lodged within the concepts derived from the careful observation of patients and within all the wisdom that has been collected over millennia—whether handed down orally or in meticulously painted characters. If there is even one chance of recovering an effective way of curing a sick person, it behooves us to leave no page unturned to find it.

Our highly technical and super-specialized era—in which a physicist and Nobel-prizewinner has to apologize five times within a few pages for treating his special subject as part of the greater realm of natural sciences—our era is in dire need of people who will dare a more expansive outlook; people who are prepared to make a bridge to that which is today discarded as superstition, but may tomorrow be recognized as scientific fact.

The history of science has taught us that many a discovery which seems ever so final, many an apparently irrevocable scientific law, will be designated incorrect or inadequate by a later generation. Let us hope that our descendants are flexible in their approach to science. For it would be a sad comment on man's intellectual progress, indeed, were he always to relegate the wisdom of the past to the realm of superstition.

If the authors have succeeded in reaching the minds of even a few of their readers—be it on a minor or a major scale—then their intentions will have been more than realized.

GLOSSARY

Aura (see *Pneuma*).

Autonomic nervous system: That nervous system which regulates bodily functions autonomously or spontaneously, i.e., cannot be controlled by our will. It is closely aligned with the hormone-forming glands. In fact, its center is situated in the cranial region near the pituitary gland. The autonomic nervous system consists of the sympathetic system—which acts mainly as the "stimulator"—and the parasympathetic system—the "preserver of the finer, constructive functions"—of the body. Both regulate the nervous control and balance of the viscera—such as heart, lungs, gut—by traveling to the organ together and interacting there—often antagonistically. Sometimes the parasympathetic nerves become the stimulators, and vice versa; for instance, the intestinal movement of contracting waves is effected by the stimulating action of the parasympathetic nerves on the smooth muscles of the gut, and the inhibiting action of the sympathetic nerves.

Chinese Philosophy: There are two major movements in Chinese philosophy: Confucianism and Taoism. The founder of Confucianism was the scholar and statesman K'ung Fu-tzu (latinized to Confucius) who lived from c. 551 to 479 B.C., an era that was marked by outbreaks of violence and extreme corruption and depravity. Confucius began in his early youth to explore the archives in search of old writings and proceeded to revise and edit those he found. His major endeavor was to study methods by which past rulers had governed, in order to find ways and means of preventing the extinction of Chinese culture and to redirect the people to the right path of life. However, he was to get much older before his teachings fell on receptive ears. He himself supposedly never put down his doctrines in writing; we owe our knowledge of him to the manuscripts written by his many disciples.

The great master's philosophy is composed of a fixed system of ethical behavior; he admonishes sovereigns and common people to live wisely—the former to rule judiciously, and the latter to pursue a moral course of life.

In sharp contrast to the tangible and practical doctrines of Confucius, the theories of his contemporary Lao-tzu are couched in the language of extremely obscure and abstract speculation. The key to Lao-tzu's mysticism is the *Wei-Wu-Wei*, the "doing by not doing," by which he does not mean "doing nothing." According to his ideas, man should be still and passive before the doings of nature, of *tao*, the "Way"; he should perform his small daily tasks and not tackle problems when they have become overwhelmingly huge. Also, people should not interfere in the politics of kings. Lao-tzu's only work—if, indeed, he wrote it himself, which is a controversial point—is the renowned *Tao Tê Ching*, in which he probes into the essence of the *tao*.

One of the major exponents of Confucianism was the philosopher Mong-tzu (born 372 B.C.), who, like his master, was accepted only after many disillusioning setbacks in his life. While Confucius' statements are sober and unadorned, Mong-tzu knows how to fascinate the reader with an elaborate and interesting style.

Especially eminent among the Taoist writers are Lieh-tzu (fl. fifth of fourth century B.C.) and Chuang-tzu (fl. fourth century B.C.). Both liked to present their ideas in the form of allegories, usually satirical. Some scholars hold that Lieh-tzu is an imaginary figure created by Chuang-tzu.

The Confucianist philosophy has been maintained in its original form and concept to this day. Taoism, on the other hand, has been transformed into a religion replete with superstition and demon-worship, and now bears hardly any traces of the genuine, original Taoism. But there are still a number of men who will withdraw from the world and live as hermits in deep and absolute seclusion, in order to contemplate the true *tao*.

A significant figure in Chinese philosophy is Mo Ti, the "philosopher of universal love." Pacifist through and through, he professed that the most essential impulse in man's life should be to approach his fellow beings with love alone. (*See also* the final chapter of this book.)

Commentaries: Ancient Chinese writings are extremely involved and vague at the same time, which has made it very difficult for later generations to read and interpret them. This deficiency gave rise to the practice of writing tome after tome of commentaries on the individual ancient works. Unfortunately, many of those cannot be read without further commentaries on the commentary.

Emodin: Constituent of many plants that have purgative properties; appears mostly in the form of a glucoside, being combined with the plant's sugar substances. It is a chemical derivative of anthraquinone, which is also the starting material for several dyestuffs (e.g., alizarine).

Exorcism: The practice of expelling evil spirits by adjuration, often by using a holy name or magic rite; the one who performs it is the exorcist (or exorciser). A vestige of this lives on in the *exsufflatio*, etc., in the baptismal rites of the Catholic Church.

Geomancy: Divination by means of figures or lines, or earth-rays, in the ground. It is used to lay out gardens, houses, and other structures, grave sites, fields, farms, etc. The instrument used is the geomantic compass, a disk with written symbols all around and a compass needle in its center. Geomancy takes into account the principles of *Yin* and *Yang* and all its ramifications and, most probably, also some very real hygienic principles.

Ginseng: Chinese: *Jen shen*, the "man-shaped root," Latin: *Panax*, belonging to the Araliaceae family. The roots of the ginseng have been esteemed as having medicinal qualities since prehistoric times.

Head's Zones (also called Head's lines, or zones of hyperalgesia): Zones of cutaneous sensitiveness associated with diseases of the viscera. Each skin zone corresponds to the organ whose nerve ends terminate in the same segment of the spinal cord as the nerve ends of the skin zone.

Huang-ti: "The Yellow Emperor." Said to have ruled from 2697 to 2595 B.C. Claimed by some to belong to the legendary period in the history of Chinese dynasties, the period from 2852 to 2205 B.C. Others list him as the founder and first ruler of the Chinese Empire. (*See also* Chapter II.)

Huang-ti Nei Ching: The Yellow Emperor's Book of Internal Medicine. It is one of the oldest medical textbooks, by many ascribed to the time of Huang-ti's reign, hence its name.

Jury Mast: A back and head support, consisting of an upright bar, the lower end of which is fixed in a spinal support made of plaster of Paris; its upper end is curved and carries a sling in which the chin and the back of the head rest.

Parasympathetic Nervous System (*see* Autonomic Nervous System).

Pneuma (literally: wind, air, spirit): The ancient Greeks believed it to be the vital soul or principle that regulates man's pulse and breathing; it is the Chinese *Ch'i*. In sense and significance, *pneuma* often cannot be distinguished from *aura* (literally: breeze, air). Both are probably best translated as "life-giving breath" or "life-giving force." In Western medicine, aura is a term applied in epilepsy. It denotes the peculiar sensation that epileptics often feel prior to a seizure; it may be a feeling of light air, or tingling, ascending from within the body or the limbs to the head, or it may be flashes of light, noises in the ear, etc. In occultism, aura refers to the form of the astral body (or astral spirit) which is allegedly visible to the persons who declare it to be so. This is obviously open to argument; but what does exist is an indefinable aura which makes it sometimes possible to recognize whether a person is really dead or not, and which has nothing to do with the so-called certain symptoms of exitus.

Predisposition: In medical terminology, a condition of special susceptibility to a disease. May be caused by lowered body-resistance, or may be genetic. Also called, especially in the latter case, disposition, or diathesis.

Psychoanalysis: A medical therapy developed by Sigmund Freud. It is based on Freud's theory that the instinctual life-impulse (id) of a human being is inhibited by education, conventions, etc., and that thereby experiences (especially internal emotional ones) are repressed into the subconscious. Freud restricted his speculations in the main to two instincts: the sex-instinct (libido) and the death-instinct (which he incorporated into his theory only later). This restriction was very early felt, even by his close disciples, to be a block to discussion of the overall issue and was eventually lifted from psychoanalysis. In principle, the cure is achieved by the patient's talking freely and without any restraint to the psychoanalyst. The patient transmits his spontaneous thoughts, association of ideas—coherent or not—and his dreams. The chance of unburdening one's mind and soul is in itself a release of tension and thus may help one to cope better with life's anxieties.

Pulse: Every time the left ventricle of the heart contracts, thereby forcing the blood through the aortic valve into the blood-vascular system, the arteries are dilated by the increased volume of blood. This creates a rhythmic wave of pulsation which extends into the finest capillaries. When this pulse-wave is measured by a pulsimeter at a certain spot (such as the usual one on the radial artery in the wrist), a definite pulse-curve will be registered, which changes according to the patient's particular condition of health or disease. By comparing this pulse-curve with the curves taken from various other spots on the patient's body, today's physician can determine several circulatory diseases.

Referred Pain: A pain that is experienced in an area remote from its actual origin, i.e., remote from the diseased part of the body. Such pain is frequent with angina pectoris, for instance, where the pain is referred into the arm. The Head's zones (q.v.) may also be considered zones of referred pain.

Sympathetic Nervous System (*see* Autonomic Nervous System).

Tao: The right Way, the primordial path and principle of nature. (*See also* Chapter I.)

Therapeutic Anesthesia: Literal translation of *Heilanästhesie;* the term as such not part of American medical terminology, although the therapy is practiced in the United States to some extent. The underlying theory of therapeutic anesthesia is the following. Pain causes defensive reactions within the organism. These reactions are often highly undesirable, if not harmful, since they tend to "trespass" into areas of the body other than that in which the disease is seated. To effect a relief of the pain will therefore contribute to a cure of the pain-causing disease. These basic, and somewhat simplified, concepts of therapeutic anesthesia have progressed considerably since their original discovery and are still being advanced. With local anesthetics (such as Novocain) results have been attained that cannot be explained by the above concepts alone. Many recent explanations seem admittedly very convincing, but have not yet been fully and scientifically accepted. (*See also* Chapter VI.)

'I HAVE SEEN THE PAST
AND IT WORKS'

By Samuel Rosen

What I have to tell is, I know, not going to be believed. I know this because a Chinese surgeon, chief at the major metropolitan hospital in Canton, told me that he had not believed it himself—until he had seen it many times over.

The scene is an operating room such as would be familiar to any surgeon American, European, or Asian. On the operating table is a vigorous man in the prime of life. He happens to be a surgeon himself. The victim of pulmonary tuberculosis, he has agreed with his colleagues that the only way to arrest his disease is to remove the upper lobe of his left lung.

Aseptic procedure is meticulous. I am gowned and masked as I would be here at Mount Sinai Hospital. So are my fellow visitors to China, the renowned cardiologists, Drs. Paul Dudley White of Boston and E. Gray Diamond of the University of Kansas School of Medicine, and our wives. Also present are the surgeon in charge, a scrub nurse and an anesthesiologist. There is one other. She is an acupuncturist.

She proceeds. She swabs the right forearm of the patient with alcohol. Then, from a variety of extremely flexible, solid, immensely fine needles immersed in alcohol, she selects one and inserts it about two centimeters into the arm, midway between wrist and elbow. The patient and his friend, the surgeon, chat amiably, while this procedure continues. The acupuncturist twirls the needle between her thumb and her first two fingers.

Twenty minutes elapse. The acupuncturist nods to the surgeon. Without the least hesitation, the surgeon takes a scalpel and swiftly cuts an incision from near the spine across the left side of the chest wall to the sternum. Then he takes a scissors-like instrument and cuts each rib away. A thoracic retractor is handed to him. He places it and exposes the chest cavity, revealing the beating heart and the collapsed lung of the patient. Meanwhile, the acupuncturist continues to twirl the needle still inserted in the patient's arm. The anesthetist is idle. The surgeon and the patient converse, and the patient drinks sips of tea from the spout of a teapot held to his mouth by a nurse.

I have seen one of the most venerable arts of Chinese traditional medicine applied in the most modern of contexts in today's China. I have seen it used, not once, but fifteen times—successfully in brain operations, thyroid adenomas, gastrectomies, laryngectomies and tonsillectomies performed in Canton, Peking and Shanghai. Each time, the standby Western-style anesthetist's skills were not needed, because this relatively new application of an ancient form of medical practice has not only replaced anesthetics but has permitted the patients, in every case to leave the operating room or the dentist's chair alert, smiling, either walking in some cases or on a stretcher in others—and waving his "Quotations from Chairman Mao Tse-tung."

In short, my American colleagues and I have seen the past and it works.

I have no explanation for this phenomenon, but science has no explanation for many observations that still elude investigation. Neither have Chinese medical men, as they frankly concede. They are investigating acupuncture anesthesia diligently, both at the basic electrophysiological level and in search for more precise definition of just which points on the human body are capable of inducing anesthesia. That the effect is present cannot be denied. Four acupuncture needles inserted in each external earlobe anesthetized a patient who then had most of his stomach removed because of a bleeding ulcer. I saw teeth extracted under the same benign influence of accurately implanted needles which were then energized either by rotation *in situ* or by inducting a weak (6-volt) direct current in each needle.

We asked what preoperative procedures were used. We were told that patients receive, as they do in this country, fifty milligrams of Demerol before surgery.

One of my colleagues asked whether Chairman Mao's "thoughts" might not have an autohypnotic or autosuggestive effect on the patient.

"Perhaps," the surgeon replied, "but we have been producing the same effects in the rabbit and the cat, and as far as we know they have not been influenced by the thought of Chairman Mao."

Dr. Samuel Rosen, Clinical Emeritus Professor of Otology at the Mount Sinai School of Medicine, and his wife visited China in 1971 as guests of the Chinese Medical Association.
I HAVE SEEN THE PAST AND IT WORKS by Samuel Rosen. Copyright © 1971 The New York Times Company. Reprinted by arrangement with The New York Times Company, New York, N. Y.

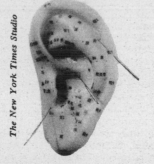

The New York Times Studio

MODEL OF AN EAR WITH ACUPUNCTURE NEEDLES.

Index